PUBLISHED BY

THE MEDICAL LETTER
on Drugs and Therapeutics

a nonprofit publication

(ISSN 0190-3454)

The Medical Letter, Inc.
1000 Main Street
New Rochelle, New York 10801-7537

800.211.2769 or 914.235.0500
FAX: 914.632.1733
www.medletter.com

OTHER PUBLICATIONS

The Medical Letter on Drugs and Therapeutics,
a bi-weekly newsletter that evaluates new drugs

Annual Bound Volume

The Medical Letter Handbook of Adverse Drug Interactions,
print and software versions

Drugs of Choice from The Medical Letter

The Medical Letter Searchable Collection 1988-2001 on CD-ROM

THE MEDICAL LETTER HANDBOOK OF ANTIMICROBIAL THERAPY
includes some material previously published in The Medical Letter

CONTENTS

Summary of Antibacterial Drugs 5

Pathogens in Specific Organs and Tissues 22

Susceptibility Tests 27

Bacterial Infections 34
  Choice of drug table 40
  Cost of oral antibacterials 53

Antimicrobial Prophylaxis in Surgery 55
  Choice of drug table 61

Prevention of Bacterial Endocarditis 64

Tuberculosis 66
  Dosage table 72

Viral Infections 74
  Dosage and cost table 84

HIV Infection 88
  HIV regimens 95
  Dosage and cost table 96
AIDS-Associated Infections: An Index 98

Sexually Transmitted Infections 99
  Choice of drug and dosage table 103

Fungal Infections 111
  Choice of drug and dosage table 111

Parasitic Infections 120

Adverse Effects 144

Dosage (with normal and decreased renal function) 160

Pregnancy, Safety 182

Trade Names 189

Index

ANTIBACTERIAL DRUGS:
A BRIEF SUMMARY FOR QUICK REFERENCE

AMINOGLYCOSIDES — Aminoglycosides are effective against many gram-negative bacteria, but not gram-positives or anaerobes. They are often used together with a β-lactam antibiotic such as ampicillin, ticarcillin, piperacillin, a cephalosporin, imipenem or aztreonam. They are ototoxic and nephrotoxic, especially in patients with diminished renal function.

Amikacin *(Amikin)* — Amikacin is often effective for treatment of infections caused by gram-negative strains resistant to gentamicin and tobramycin, including some strains of *Pseudomonas aeruginosa* and *Acinetobacter*. It is generally reserved for treatment of serious infections caused by amikacin-susceptible gram-negative bacteria known or suspected to be resistant to the other aminoglycosides. Like other aminoglycosides, its distribution to the lungs is limited and when used to treat gram-negative bacilli that cause pneumonia it should be combined with another agent to which the organism is susceptible, such as a β-lactam. It has also been used concurrently with other drugs for treatment of some mycobacterial infections.

Gentamicin (*Garamycin*, and others) — Useful for treatment of many hospital-acquired infections caused by gram-negative bacteria. Strains of gram-negative bacilli resistant to gentamicin are often susceptible to amikacin or to one of the third-generation cephalosporins, cefepime, or imipenem or meropenem. Gentamicin is also used with penicillin G, ampicillin or vancomycin for treatment of endocarditis caused by susceptible enterococci.

Kanamycin (*Kantrex*, and others) — Active against some gram-negative bacilli (except *Pseudomonas* or anaerobes), but most centers now use gentamicin, tobramycin or amikacin instead. Kanamycin can be useful concurrently with other drugs for treatment of tuberculosis.

Neomycin (many manufacturers) — A drug that can cause severe damage to hearing and renal function and has the same antibacterial spectrum as kanamycin. Parenteral formulations have no rational use because of their toxicity. Deafness has also followed topical use over large areas of skin, injection into cavities such as joints, and oral administration, especially in patients with renal insufficiency.

Streptomycin — Streptomycin has been displaced by gentamicin for treatment of gram-negative infections, but it is still sometimes used concurrently with other drugs for treatment of tuberculosis and is occasionally used with penicillin, ampicillin or vancomycin to treat enterococcal endocarditis.

Tobramycin (*Nebcin*, and others) — Similar to gentamicin but with greater activity *in vitro* against *Pseudomonas aeruginosa* and less activity against *Serratia*. In clinical use, it is not certain that it is significantly less nephrotoxic than gentamicin.

AMINOSALICYLIC ACID (PAS) — Used in antituberculosis regimens for many years, its distressing gastrointestinal effects caused many patients to stop taking it prematurely. An enteric-coated oral formulation *(Paser)* is more tolerable, and is used occasionally in combination with other drugs in treating tuberculosis due to organisms resistant to first-line drugs.

AMOXICILLIN (*Amoxil*, and others) — An oral semisynthetic penicillin similar to ampicillin, it is better absorbed and may cause less diarrhea. Amoxicillin is at least as effective as oral ampicillin for the treatment of most infections, with the exception of shigellosis.

AMOXICILLIN/CLAVULANIC ACID *(Augmentin)* — The β-lactamase inhibitor, potassium clavulanate, extends amoxicillin's spectrum of activity to include β-lactamase-producing strains of *Staphylococcus aureus, Haemophilus influenzae, Moraxella catarrhalis* and many strains of enteric gram-negative bacilli, including anaerobes such as *Bacteroides* spp. This combination may be useful for oral treatment of bite wounds, otitis media, sinusitis and some lower respiratory tract and urinary tract infections, but it can cause a higher incidence of diarrhea and other gastrointestinal symptoms than amoxicillin alone, and less costly alternatives are available.

AMPICILLIN (*Principen*, and others) — This semisynthetic penicillin is as effective as penicillin G in pneumococcal, streptococcal and meningococcal infections, and is also active against some strains of *Salmonella, Shigella, Escherichia coli* and *Haemophilus influenzae* and many strains of *Proteus mirabilis*. The drug is not effective against penicillinase-producing staphylococci or β-lactamase-producing gram-negative bacteria. Rashes are more frequent with ampicillin than with other penicillins.

AMPICILLIN/SULBACTAM *(Unasyn)* — A parenteral combination of ampicillin with the β-lactamase inhibitor sulbactam, which extends the antibacterial spectrum of ampicillin to include β-lactamase-producing strains of *Staphylococcus aureus, Haemophilus influenzae, Moraxella catarrhalis, Neisseria* and many gram-negative bacilli, including *Bacteroides fragilis*, but not *Pseudomonas aeruginosa, Enterobacter* or *Serratia*. It may be useful for treatment of gynecological and intra-abdominal infections. Some strains of *Acinetobacter* resistant to all other antibiotics may respond to high doses of ampicillin/sulbactam in combination with polymyxins.

AZITHROMYCIN *(Zithromax)* — See Macrolides

AZTREONAM *(Azactam)* — A parenteral β-lactam antibiotic active against most aerobic gram-negative bacilli, including *Pseudomonas aeruginosa*, but not against gram-positive organisms or anaerobes. Aztreonam has little cross-allergenicity with penicillins and cephalosporins.

BACITRACIN — A nephrotoxic drug used in the past to treat severe systemic infections caused by staphylococci resistant to penicillin G. Its use is now restricted mainly to topical application.

CAPREOMYCIN *(Capastat)* — A second-line antituberculosis drug

CARBAPENEMS

Ertapenem (*Invanz* – Medical Letter 2002; 44:25) — A new parenteral carbapenem with a longer half-life but narrower antibacterial spectrum than imipenem and meropenem. It is more active against some extended-spectrum β-lactamase-producing gram-negative bacilli, but less active against gram-positive cocci, *Pseudomonas aeruginosa* and *Acinetobacter* spp. For empiric treatment of intra-abdominal, pelvic and urinary tract infections and community-acquired pneumonia, it offers no clear advantage over older drugs.

Imipenem/Cilastatin *(Primaxin)* — A parenteral β-lactam with an especially broad antibacterial spectrum. Cilastatin sodium inhibits renal tubular metabolism of imipenem. This combination may be especially useful for treatment of serious infections in which aerobic gram-negative bacilli, anaerobes, and *Staphylococcus aureus* might all be involved. It is active against many gram-negative bacilli that are resistant to third- and fourth-generation cephalosporins, aztreonam and aminoglycosides. Resistance to imipenem in *Pseudomonas aeruginosa* occasionally develops during therapy.

Meropenem *(Merrem)* — A carbapenem for parenteral use similar to imipenem/cilastatin. It may have less potential than imipenem for causing seizures.

CARBENICILLIN *(Geocillin)* —The oral indanyl ester of carbenicillin; it does not produce therapeutic blood levels, but can be used for treatment of urinary tract infections, including those due to susceptible gram-negative bacilli such as *Pseudomonas aeruginosa* that may be resistant to other drugs.

CEPHALOSPORINS — All cephalosporins are active against most gram-positive cocci, and many strains of gram-negative bacilli. These drugs are often prescribed for patients allergic to penicillin, but such patients may also have allergic reactions to cephalosporins.

The cephalosporins can be classified into four "generations" based on their activity against gram-negative organisms. All first-generation drugs have a similar spectrum, including many gram-positive cocci (but not enterococci or methicillin-resistant *Staphylococcus aureus*), *Escherichia coli, Klebsiella pneumoniae,* and *Proteus mirabilis.* Among the first-generation parenteral cephalosporins, **cefazolin** (*Ancef,* and others) is less painful on intramuscular injection than **cephapirin** (*Cefadyl,* and others). The first-generation parenteral cephalosporins are usually given intravenously, and cefazolin is most frequently used because of its longer half-life.

The second-generation cephalosporins have broader *in vitro* activity against gram-negative bacteria. **Cefamandole** *(Mandol)* has increased activity against *Haemophilus influenzae* and some gram-negative bacilli, but is occasionally associated with prothrombin deficiency and bleeding. **Cefoxitin** *(Mefoxin)* has improved activity against *Bacteroides fragilis, Neisseria gonorrhoeae* and some aerobic gram-negative bacilli. **Cefotetan** *(Cefotan)* has a spectrum of activity similar to that of cefoxitin; it has a side chain that, with other cephalosporins, has rarely been associated with prothrombin deficiency and bleeding. **Cefuroxime** *(Zinacef, Kefurox)*, another second-generation cephalosporin, has a spectrum of activity similar to cefamandole. Cefuroxime and cefamandole are less active than third-generation cephalosporins against penicillin-resistant strains of *Streptococcus pneumoniae.* **Cefonicid** *(Monocid)* has a longer half-life than the other second-generation cephalosporins, but is less active against gram-positive organisms and less active than cefoxitin against anaerobes.

The third-generation cephalosporins, **cefotaxime** *(Claforan)*, **cefoperazone** *(Cefobid)*, **ceftizoxime** *(Cefizox)*, **ceftriaxone** *(Rocephin)* and **ceftazidime** (*Fortaz,* and others), and the fourth-generation cephalosporin, **cefepime** *(Maxipime*), are more active than the second-generation cephalosporins against enteric gram-negative bacilli, including nosocomially acquired strains resistant to multiple antibiotics. These agents are highly active against *Haemophilus influenzae* and *Neisseria gonorrhoeae,* including penicillinase-producing strains. Except for ceftazidime, they are moderately active against anaerobes, but often less so than metronidazole, chloramphenicol, clindamycin, cefoxitin, cefotetan, piperacillin/tazobactam, ticarcillin/clavulanic acid, or carbapenems. Ceftazidime has poor activity against gram-positive organisms and anaerobes. Cefotaxime, ceftizoxime, ceftriaxone and cefepime are the most active *in vitro* against gram-positive organisms, but ceftizoxime has poor activity against *Streptococcus pneumoniae* that are intermediate or highly resistant to penicillin. Cefoperazone, which can cause bleeding, is less active than other third-generation cephalosporins against many gram-negative bacilli, but more active than cefotaxime, ceftizoxime or ceftriaxone against *Pseudomonas.* Ceftazidime and cefepime have the greatest activity among the cephalosporins against *Pseudomonas.* Cefepime has somewhat greater activity against enteric gram-negative bacilli than the third-generation cephalosporins.

The third-generation cephalosporins and cefepime are expensive, but are useful for treatment of serious hospital-associated gram-negative infections when used alone or in combination with aminoglycosides such as gentamicin, tobramycin or amikacin. However, gram-negative bacilli that produce extended spectrum β-lactamases, particularly some *Klebsiella* strains and those that produce chromosomally-encoded β-lactamases, are resistant to third-generation cephalosporins. These organisms are often hospital-associated. Cefipime may be more active than the third-generation cephalosporin against these strains, but imipenem, meropenem and ertapenem are most consistently active against them. Cefotaxime and ceftriaxone are often used for treatment of meningitis. Ceftriaxone has been widely used for single-dose treatment of gonorrhea. All cephalosporins are inactive against enterococci and methicillin-resistant staphylococci.

Cephalexin (*Keflex,* and others), **cephradine** (*Velosef,* and others), and **cefadroxil** (*Duricef,* and others) are well-absorbed oral cephalosporins with first-generation antimicrobial activity; cephradine is also available for parenteral use. **Cefaclor** (*Ceclor,* and others), **cefuroxime axetil** *(Ceftin)*, **cefprozil** *(Cefzil)* and **loracarbef** *(Lorabid)* are oral second-generation agents with increased activity against *Haemophilus influenzae* and *Moraxella catarrhalis*. **Cefixime** *(Suprax)* is an oral cephalosporin with activity against gram-positive organisms similar to that of first-generation cephalosporins except for its poor activity against staphylococci; against gram-negative bacteria, it has greater activity than second-generation cephalosporins. It is recommended for single-dose oral treatment of gonorrhea. **Cefpodoxime proxetil** *(Vantin)*, **cefdinir** *(Omnicef)* and **cefditoren pivoxil** (*Spectracef* – Medical Letter 2002; 44:5) are oral cephalosporins similar to cefixime, but with greater activity against methicillin-susceptible staphylococci. **Ceftibuten** *(Cedax)* is an oral cephalosporin similar to cefixime in its gram-negative activity and poor activity against staphylococci, but it has only inconsistent activity against *Streptococcus pneumoniae*.

CHLORAMPHENICOL (*Chloromycetin,* and others) — An effective drug for treatment of meningitis, epiglottitis, or other serious infections caused by *Haemophilus influenzae,* severe infections with *Salmonella typhi,* for some severe infections caused by *Bacteroides* (especially those in the central nervous system), and for treatment of vancomycin-resistant *Enterococcus*. Chloramphenicol is often an effective alternative for treatment of pneumococcal or meningococcal meningitis in patients allergic to penicillin, but some strains of *Streptococcus pneumoniae* are resistant to it. Because it can cause fatal blood dyscrasias, chloramphenicol should be used only for serious infections caused by susceptible bacteria that cannot be treated effectively with less toxic agents.

CINOXACIN (*Cinobac*, and others) — See Quinolones

CIPROFLOXACIN *(Cipro)* — See Fluoroquinolones

CLARITHROMYCIN *(Biaxin)* — See Macrolides

CLINDAMYCIN (*Cleocin*, and others) — A derivative of lincomycin with a similar antibacterial spectrum, clindamycin can cause severe diarrhea and pseudomembranous colitis. It is one of the alternative drugs for anaerobic infections outside the central nervous system, and can also be used as an alternative for treatment of some staphylococcal infections in patients allergic to penicillins. Clindamycin is also used concurrently with other drugs to treat *Pneumocystis carinii* pneumonia and toxoplasmosis. Clindamycin may be beneficial in treatment of necrotizing fasciitis due to Group A streptococcus but, because of the possibility of resistance to clindamycin, it should be used in combination with penicillin G.

CLOFAZIMINE *(Lamprene)* — An oral agent used with other drugs for treatment of leprosy.

CLOXACILLIN — See Penicillinase-resistant Penicillins

COLISTIMETHATE *(Coly-Mycin)* — See Polymyxins

CYCLOSERINE (*Seromycin*, and others) — A second-line antituberculosis drug.

DEMECLOCYCLINE *(Declomycin)* — See Tetracyclines

DICLOXACILLIN (*Dycill*, and others) — See Penicillinase-resistant Penicillins

DIRITHROMYCIN *(Dynabac)* — See Macrolides

DOXYCYCLINE *(Vibramycin*, and others) — See Tetracyclines

ENOXACIN *(Penetrex)* — See Fluoroquinolones

ERTAPENEM *(Invanz)* — See Carbapenems

ERYTHROMYCIN (*Erythrocin*, and others) — See Macrolides

ERYTHROMYCIN-SULFISOXAZOLE *(Pediazole*, and others) — See Macrolides

ETHIONAMIDE *(Trecator-SC)* — A second-line antituberculosis drug.

ETHAMBUTOL *(Myambutol)* — Often used in antituberculosis regimens, it can cause optic neuritis.

FLUOROQUINOLONES — With the increased use of fluoroquinolones, resistant organisms have become more frequent, especially among strains of *Staphylococcus aureus* and *Pseudomonas aeruginosa*. Resistance among *Streptococcus pneumoniae* strains has begun to emerge but is still rare, especially in the US. None of these agents is recommended for use in children or pregnant women.

Ciprofloxacin *(Cipro)* — Used for oral or intravenous treatment of a wide variety of gram-positive and gram-negative bacterial infections in adults, including those due to methicillin-susceptible and methicillin-resistant staphylococci, *Haemophilus influenzae, Neisseria,* enteric pathogens and other aerobic gram-negative bacilli, and *Pseudomonas aeruginosa*, but not anaerobes. Ciprofloxacin is now the preferred prophylactic agent for contacts of patients with meningococcal disease. It is also used for prophylaxis after *Bacillus antracis* (Anthrax) exposure. For treatment of *Mycobacterium avium* and *M. tuberculosis* infections, it is effective in combination with other drugs. Emergence of resistance in staphylococcal and *Pseudomonas* strains and other gram-negative organisms is increasingly encountered, and central-nervous-system toxicity occurs occasionally.

Enoxacin *(Penetrex)* — An oral fluoroquinolone similar to ciprofloxacin that can be used to treat urinary tract infection and uncomplicated gonorrhea.

Gatifloxacin *(Tequin)*, **levofloxacin** *(Levaquin)*, and **moxifloxacin** *(Avelox)* — More active than ciprofloxacin or ofloxacin against gram-positive organisms, such as *Streptococcus pneumoniae,* including strains highly resistant to penicillin, and *Staphylococcus aureus.* Like other fluoroquinolones, they are active against *Legionella pneumophila, Chlamydia spp., Mycoplasma pneumoniae, Haemophilus influenzae* and *Moraxella catarrhalis.* All are effective for many community-acquired respiratory infections and are available for both oral and parenteral use.

Lomefloxacin *(Maxaquin)* — An oral once-a-day fluoroquinolone promoted for treatment of urinary tract infections and bronchitis, but pneumococci and other streptococci are resistant to the drug.

Norfloxacin *(Noroxin)* — An oral fluoroquinolone for treatment of urinary tract infections due to Enterobacteriaceae, *Enterococcus* or *Pseudomonas aeruginosa.*

Ofloxacin *(Floxin)* — An oral and intravenous fluoroquinolone similar to ciprofloxacin but less active against *Pseudomonas.* Ofloxacin can be used for single-dose treatment of gonorrhea and for seven-day treatment of chlamydial infections.

Trovafloxacin *(Trovan)* has been associated with rare but fatal hepatitis, and should be restricted to brief (<14 days) inpatient use with liver monitoring.

FOSFOMYCIN *(Monurol)* — Can be used as a single-dose oral agent with moderate effectiveness for treatment of uncomplicated urinary tract infections caused by many strains of enteric gram-negative bacilli, enterococci and some strains of *Staphylococcus saphrophyticus,* but generally not *Pseudomonas.* It is much more expensive than trimethoprim/sulfamethoxazole.

FURAZOLIDONE *(Furoxone)* — An oral nonabsorbable antimicrobial agent of the nitrofuran group that inhibits monoamine oxidase (MAO). The manufacturer recommends it for treatment of bacterial diarrhea. Its safety has been questioned (oral administration induces mammary tumors in rats) and other more effective drugs are available.

GATIFLOXACIN *(Tequin)* — See Fluoroquinolones

GENTAMICIN *(Garamycin,* and others) — See Aminoglycosides

IMIPENEM/CILASTATIN *(Primaxin)* — See Carbapenems

ISONIAZID (*Nydrazid,* and others) — A major antituberculosis drug that can cause fatal hepatitis. **Rifampin-isoniazid-pyrazinamide** *(Rifater)* and **rifampin-isoniazid** *(Rifamate)* are fixed-dose combinations for treatment of tuberculosis.

KANAMYCIN (*Kantrex,* and others) — See Aminoglycosides

LEVOFLOXACIN *(Levaquin)* — See Fluoroquinolones

LINCOMYCIN *(Lincocin)* — Similar to clindamycin in antibacterial activity and adverse effects. Rarely indicated for treatment of any infection because it is less active than clindamycin.

LINEZOLID (*Zyvox* – Medical Letter 2000; 42:45) — An oxazolidinone antibiotic available in both an oral and intravenous formulation. It is active against *Enterococcus faecium* and *E. faecalis* including vancomycin-resistant enterococcal infections. Linezolid is also active against methicillin-resistant *Staphylococcus aureus, S. epidermidis* and penicillin-resistant *Streptococcus pneumoniae.* Reversible thrombocytopenia has occurred, especially with therapy for more than 2 weeks. Emergence of resistance has been observed with enterococcal strains.

LOMEFLOXACIN *(Maxaquin)* — See Fluoroquinolones

MACROLIDES

Azithromycin *(Zithromax)* — A macrolide antibiotic that has much less gastrointestinal toxicity than erythromycin. A single dose has been effective for treatment of urethritis and cervicitis caused by *Chlamydia.* Azithromycin is useful in treating *Mycoplasma pneumoniae, Chlamydia pneumoniae* and *Legionella pneumophila* pneumonias, as well as some respiratory infections due to *Streptococcus pneumoniae, Haemophilus influenzae* or *Moraxella catarrhalis.* However, an increasing number of *S. pneumoniae* strains have become resistant to the macrolides. Azithromycin alone is effective for prevention of *Mycobacterium avium* infections, and combined with other drugs, such as ethambutol, rifabutin or ciprofloxacin, it is effective for treatment.

Clarithromycin *(Biaxin)* — A macrolide antibiotic similar to azithromycin, but with a shorter half-life. It is somewhat more active than azithromycin against gram-positive organisms and less active against gram-negative organisms. Clarithromycin is effective for prevention of *Mycobacterium avium* infections and, combined with other drugs, for treatment of both *M. avium* and *Helicobacter pylori.* It has fewer adverse effects than azithromycin, but more adverse drug interactions (*Medical Letter Handbook of Adverse Drug Interactions* 2002, page 350).

Dirithromycin *(Dynabac)* — Similar to erythromycin; it can be given once a day.

Erythromycin (*Erythrocin,* and others) — Used especially for respiratory tract infections due to pneumococci or Group A streptococci in patients allergic to penicillin, for pneumonia due to *Mycoplasma pneumoniae* or *Chlamydia spp.,* and for treatment of infection caused by *Legionella pneumophila,* erythromycin has few adverse effects except for frequent gastrointestinal disturbances and some drug interactions (*Medical Letter Handbook of Adverse Drug Interactions,* 2002, page 350). The estolate formulation *(Ilosone)* can cause cholestatic jaundice. Erythromycin is not recommended for treatment of serious staphylococcal infections, even when the organisms are susceptible to the drug *in vitro,* because of rapid development of resistance. Strains of *Streptococcus pneumoniae* and Group A streptococci resistant to erythromycin have become more frequent.

Erythromycin/Sulfisoxazole (*Pediazole,* and others) — A combination of 100 mg of erythromycin ethylsuccinate and 300 mg sulfisoxazole acetyl per half-teaspoon for oral treatment of acute otitis media.

Troleandomycin *(TAO)* — This oral drug has an antibacterial spectrum like that of the erythromycins, but it can cause cholestatic jaundice, and there are no reasonable indications for its use.

MEROPENEM *(Merrem)* — See Carbapenems

METHENAMINES (*Mandelamine*, and others) — Oral drugs that can sterilize an acid urine. They are used for prophylaxis of chronic or recurrent urinary tract infections, but trimethoprim/sulfamethoxazole is more effective.

METHICILLIN — See Penicillinase-resistant Penicillins

METRONIDAZOLE (*Flagyl*, and others) — Available in oral form for treatment of trichomoniasis, amebiasis, giardiasis and *Gardnerella vaginalis* vaginitis, metronidazole is also available for intravenous treatment of anaerobic bacterial infections. Good penetration of the blood-brain barrier may be an advantage in treating central-nervous-system infections due to *Bacteroides fragilis.* Metronidazole is also used to treat pseudomembranous enterocolitis due to *Clostridium difficile.*

MINOCYCLINE (*Minocin*, and others) — See Tetracyclines

MOXIFLOXACIN *(Avelox)* — See Fluoroquinolones

NAFCILLIN (*Nafcil*, and others) — See Penicillinase-resistant Penicillins

NALIDIXIC ACID (*NegGram*, and others) — See Quinolones

NEOMYCIN (many manufacturers) — See Aminoglycosides

NITROFURANTOIN (*Macrodantin*, and others) — This oral agent is used for prophylaxis or treatment of urinary tract infections. Because of its potential toxicity, nitrofurantoin should not be used when renal function is markedly diminished. Nausea and vomiting are often troublesome, and peripheral neuropathy, pulmonary reactions and severe hepatotoxicity may occur.

NORFLOXACIN *(Noroxin)* — See Fluoroquinolones

OFLOXACIN *(Floxin)* — See Fluoroquinolones

OXACILLIN — See Penicillinase-resistant Penicillins

PENICILLIN — Penicillin remains the drug of choice for Group A streptococcal infections and for the treatment of syphilis and some other infections. Clindamycin may be beneficial for treatment of Group A streptococcal necrotizing fasciitis, but it should be combined with penicillin G because of increasing resistance to clindamycin in Group A streptococcus. *Streptococcus pneumoniae* strains frequently show intermediate or high-level resistance to penicillin. Penicillin is the drug of choice for fully sensitive strains, and high doses of penicillin, cefotaxime or ceftriaxone are effective for pneumonia due to strains with intermediate sensitivity, but vancomycin is recommended for highly resistant strains, especially for meningitis.

PENICILLINASE-RESISTANT PENICILLINS — The drugs of choice for treatment of infections caused by penicillinase-producing staphylococci, they are also effective against penicillin-sensitive pneumococci and Group A streptococci. For oral use, **cloxacillin** or **dicloxacillin** is preferred; for severe infections, a parenteral formulation of **nafcillin** or **oxacillin** should be used. **Methicillin** is no longer marketed in the US. Strains of *Staphylococcus aureus* or *epidermidis* that are resistant to these penicillins ("methicillin-resistant") are also resistant to cephalosporins, and carbapenems. Infections caused by these strains should be treated with vancomycin, with or without rifampin and/or gentamicin. Neither ampicillin, amoxicillin, carbenicillin, piperacillin nor ticarcillin is effective against penicillinase-producing staphylococci.

PIPERACILLIN *(Pipracil)* — A penicillin for parenteral treatment of gram-negative bacillary infections. It is similar to ticarcillin in antibacterial activity, but covers a wider spectrum, particularly against *Klebsiella pneumoniae* and *Bacteroides fragilis*. Its *in vitro* activity against *Pseudomonas* is greater than that of ticarcillin, but increased clinical effectiveness in *Pseudomonas* infections has not been demonstrated. Piperacillin is also active against some gram-positive cocci, including streptococci and some strains of *Enterococcus*. For treatment of serious gram-negative infections, it should generally be used in combination with an aminoglycoside such as gentamicin, tobramycin or amikacin.

PIPERACILLIN/TAZOBACTAM *(Zosyn)* — A parenteral formulation combining piperacillin with tazobactam, a β-lactamase-inhibitor. The addition of the β-lactamase inhibitor extends the spectrum of piperacillin to include β-lactamase producing strains of staphylococci and many gram-negative bacilli, including *Bacteroides fragilis*. The combination of the two drugs is no more active against *Pseudomonas aeruginosa* than piperacillin alone.

POLYMYXINS B AND E (polymyxin B – various generics; polymyxin E – *Coly-Mycin*; colistimethate; colistin sulfate) — The polymyxins are used topically in combination with other antibiotics for treatment of infected wounds and otitis externa. They should generally not be used parenterally because safer and more effective alternatives are available. However, some strains of *Acinetobacter* are resistant to all other available antibiotics and infections due to those strains have been treated with polymyxin, sometimes combined with high doses of sulbactam (in the form of ampicillin/sulbactam), with some reports of benefit.

PYRAZINAMIDE — An antituberculosis drug now often used in the initial treatment regimen. Rifampin-isoniazid-pyrazinamide *(Rifater)* is a fixed-dose combination for treatment of tuberculosis.

QUINOLONES

Nalidixic Acid (*NegGram*, and others) — An oral drug active *in vitro* against many gram-negative organisms that commonly cause urinary tract infections. Development of resistance by initially susceptible strains is rapid, however, and clinical results are much less favorable than would be expected from sensitivity testing alone. Nalidixic acid can cause severe adverse effects, including visual disturbances, intracranial hypertension, and convulsions. Other drugs are generally preferred for treatment of urinary tract infections.

Cinoxacin (*Cinobac*, and others) — An oral drug similar to nalidixic acid for treatment of urinary tract infections.

QUINUPRISTIN/DALFOPRISTIN — Two streptogramin antibacterials marketed in a fixed-dose combination *(Synercid)* for parenteral use (Medical Letter 1999; 41:109). The combination is active against vancomycin-resistant *Enterococcus faecium* (but not *E. faecalis*) as well as *Staphylococcus aureus, Streptococcus pneumoniae* and *S. pyogenes*. Adverse effects include frequent thrombophlebitis at the infusion site (it is best given through a central venous catheter) and arthralgias and myalgias. Medical Letter consultants suggest that its use be restricted to treatment of vancomycin-resistant *E. faecium* infections; use in treating other gram-positive bacterial infections should be limited to those for which other drugs are ineffective or not tolerable.

RIFABUTIN *(Mycobutin)* — Similar to rifampin, rifabutin is used to prevent and treat tuberculosis and disseminated *Mycobacterium avium* infections in patients with AIDS. It has fewer drug interactions than rifampin.

RIFAMPIN *(Rifadin, Rimactane)* — A major drug for treatment of tuberculosis. To prevent emergence of resistant organisms, it should be used together with other antituberculosis drugs. It is sometimes used concurrently with other drugs for treatment of *Mycobacterium avium* infections in AIDS patients. Rifampin is also useful for prophylaxis in close contacts of patients with sulfonamide-resistant meningococcal disease and for prophylaxis in children who are close contacts of patients with *Haemophilus influenzae* meningitis. **Rifampin-isoniazid-pyrazinamide** *(Rifater)* and **rifampin-isoniazid** *(Rifamate)* are fixed-dose combinations for treatment of tuberculosis.

RIFAPENTINE *(Priftin)* — A long-acting analog of rifampin used in the treatment of tuberculosis. Studies of its effectiveness are limited. Until more data become available, rifampin is preferred.

SPECTINOMYCIN *(Trobicin)* — A single-dose alternative for treatment of urogenital or anal gonorrhea. It is effective for penicillin-resistant infections and for patients who are allergic to penicillin. Spectinomycin is not effective against syphilis.

STREPTOMYCIN — See Aminoglycosides

SULFONAMIDES — The main use of sulfonamides is for treatment of acute, uncomplicated urinary tract infections. A soluble oral sulfonamide such as sulfisoxazole (*Gantrisin*, and others) is preferred.

TETRACYCLINES — Doxycycline, oxytetracycline *(Terramycin)*, and **minocycline** are available in both oral and parenteral formulations; **tetracycline** and **demeclocycline** *(Declomycin)* are available only for oral use. Parenteral tetracyclines can cause severe liver damage, especially when given to patients with diminished renal function. **Doxycycline** (*Vibramycin*, and others) requires fewer doses and causes less gastrointestinal disturbance than other tetracyclines. It can be used for prophylaxis after *Bacillus anthracis* (anthrax) exposure. **Minocycline** (*Minocin*, and others) may be useful for prophylactic treatment of close contacts of patients with meningococcal infection, but it frequently causes vomiting and vertigo.

TICARCILLIN *(Ticar)* — A penicillin similar to carbenicillin. Large parenteral doses of this semisynthetic penicillin can cure serious infections caused by susceptible strains of *Pseudomonas, Proteus* and some other gram-negative organisms. *Klebsiella* are generally resistant. Ticarcillin is also active against some gram-positive cocci, including streptococci and some strains of *Enterococcus*. It is often given together with another drug such as gentamicin, tobramycin or amikacin for treatment of serious systemic infections. It is less active than ampicillin, amoxicillin or piperacillin against strains of *Streptococcus pneumoniae* with reduced susceptibility to penicillin and against enterococci.

TICARCILLIN/CLAVULANIC ACID *(Timentin)* — A parenteral preparation combining ticarcillin with potassium clavulanate, a β-lactamase inhibitor. The addition of the β-lactamase inhibitor extends the antibacterial spectrum of ticarcillin to include β-lactamase producing strains of *Staphylococcus aureus, Haemophilus influenzae*, and enteric gram-negative bacilli, including *Bacteroides fragilis*. The combination is no more active against *Pseudomonas aeruginosa* than ticarcillin alone.

TOBRAMYCIN (*Nebcin*, and others) — See Aminoglycosides

TRIMETHOPRIM (*Proloprim*, and others) — An agent marketed only for oral treatment of uncomplicated urinary tract infections caused by gram-negative bacilli. Frequent use has the potential for producing organisms resistant not only to this drug but also to trimethoprim/sulfamethoxazole.

TRIMETHOPRIM/SULFAMETHOXAZOLE (*Bactrim, Septra,* and others) — A combination of a folic acid antagonist and a sulfonamide, useful especially for oral treatment of urinary tract infections, shigellosis, otitis media, travelers' diarrhea, bronchitis, and *Pneumocystis carinii* pneumonia. An intravenous preparation is available for treatment of serious infections.

TROLEANDOMYCIN *(TAO)* — See Macrolides

TROVAFLOXACIN *(Trovan)* — See Fluoroquinolones

VANCOMYCIN (*Vancocin,* and others) — An effective alternative to the penicillins for endocarditis caused by *Streptococcus viridans* or *Enterococcus,* for severe staphylococcal infections, and for penicillin-resistant *S. pneumococcus* infections. An increasing number of strains of enterococci, however, are resistant to vancomycin. Vancomycin is the drug of choice for treatment of infections caused by methicillin-resistant *Staphylococcus aureus* and *epidermidis,* but for strains that are methicillin-sensitive, nafcillin or oxacillin is more effective. Oral treatment with vancomycin is effective in treating antibiotic-associated colitis due to *Clostridium difficile,* but metronidazole is generally preferred because the increasing use of oral vancomycin has probably promoted the emergence of vancomycin-resistant enterococci.

PATHOGENS MOST LIKELY TO CAUSE INFECTIONS IN SPECIFIC ORGANS AND TISSUES

In many acute and most chronic infections, the choice of antimicrobial therapy can await the results of appropriate cultures and antimicrobial susceptibility tests. In acute life-threatening infections such as meningitis, pneumonia or bacteremia, however, and in other infections that have reached a serious stage, waiting 24 to 48 hours can be dangerous, and the choice of an antimicrobial agent for initial use must be based on tentative identification of the pathogen. Knowing the organisms most likely to cause infection in specific tissues, together with evaluation of gram-stained smears and familiarity with the antimicrobial susceptibility patterns of organisms prevalent in the hospital or community, permits a rational choice of initial treatment.

In the table below, bacteria, fungi and some viruses are listed in estimated order of the frequency with which they cause acute infection, but these frequencies are subject to annual, seasonal and geographical variation. The order of pathogens may also vary depending on whether the infections are community or hospital-acquired, and whether the patient is immunosuppressed or not. This listing is based both on published reports and on the experience of Medical Letter consultants. Organisms not listed here may also be important causes of infection.

TABLE OF BACTERIA, FUNGI, AND SOME VIRUSES MOST LIKELY TO CAUSE ACUTE INFECTIONS

BLOOD (SEPTICEMIA) Newborn Infants

1. *Streptococcus* Group B
2. *Escherichia coli* (or other gram-negative bacilli)
3. *Listeria monocytogenes*
4. *Staphylococcus aureus*
5. *Streptococcus pyogenes* (Group A)
6. *Enterococcus*
7. *Streptococcus pneumoniae*

Children

1. *Streptococcus pneumoniae*
2. *Neisseria meningitidis*
3. *Staphylococcus aureus*
4. *Streptococcus pyogenes* (Group A)
5. *Haemophilus influenzae*
6. *Escherichia coli* (or other gram-negative bacilli)

Adults

1. *Escherichia coli* (or other enteric gram-negative bacilli)
2. *Staphylococcus aureus*
3. *Streptococcus pneumoniae*

Adults *(continued)*

4. *Enterococcus*
5. Non-enteric gram-negative bacilli *(Pseudomonas, Acinetobacter, Aeromonas)*
6. *Candida* spp. and other fungi
7. *Staphylococcus epidermidis*
8. *Streptococcus pyogenes* (Group A)
9. Other streptococci (non-Group A and not Lancefield-groupable)
10. *Bacteroides*
11. *Neisseria meningitidis*
12. *Neisseria gonorrhoeae*
13. *Fusobacterium*
14. Mycobacteria
15. *Rickettsia*
16. *Ehrlichia* spp.
17. *Brucella* spp.
18. *Leptospira*

MENINGES

1. Viruses (enterovirus, mumps, herpes simplex, HIV, arbovirus and others)
2. *Neisseria meningitidis*
3. *Streptococcus pneumoniae*
4. *Streptococcus* Group B (infants less than two months old)
5. *Escherichia coli* (or other gram-negative bacilli)
6. *Haemophilus influenzae* (in children)
7. *Streptococcus pyogenes* (Group A)
8. *Staphylococcus aureus* (with endocarditis or after neurosurgery, brain abscess)
9. *Mycobacterium tuberculosis*
10. *Cryptococcus neoformans* and other fungi
11. *Listeria monocytogenes*
12. *Enterococcus* (neonatal period)
13. *Treponema pallidum*
14. *Leptospira*
15. *Borrelia burgdorferi*
16. *Toxoplasma gondii**

BRAIN AND PERIMENINGEAL SPACES

1. Herpes simplex (encephalitis)
2. Anaerobic streptococci and/or *Bacteroides* (cerebritis, brain abscess, and subdural empyema)
3. *Staphylococcus aureus* (cerebritis, brain abscess, epidural abscess)
4. *Haemophilus influenzae* (subdural empyema)
5. *Arbovirus* (encephalitis)
6. Mumps (encephalitis)
7. *Toxoplasma gondii** (encephalitis)
8. Human immunodeficiency virus (HIV)
9. *Mycobacterium tuberculosis*
10. *Nocardia* (brain abscess)
11. *Listeria monocytogenes* (encephalitis)
12. *Treponema pallidum*
13. *Cryptococcus neoformans* and other fungi
14. *Borrelia burgdorferi*

ENDOCARDIUM

1. Viridans group of *Streptococcus*
2. *Enterococcus*
3. *Staphylococcus aureus*
4. *Streptococcus bovis*
5. *Staphylococcus epidermidis*
6. *Candida albicans* and other fungi
7. Gram-negative bacilli
8. *Streptococcus pneumoniae*
9. *Streptococcus pyogenes* (Group A)
10. *Corynebacterium* (especially with prosthetic valves)
11. *Haemophilus, Actinobacillus,* or *Cardiobacterium hominis*

BONES (OSTEOMYELITIS)

1. *Staphylococcus aureus*
2. *Salmonella* (or other gram-negative bacilli)
3. *Streptococcus pyogenes* (Group A)
4. *Mycobacterium tuberculosis*
5. Anaerobic streptococci (chronic)
6. *Bacteroides* (chronic)

JOINTS

1. *Staphylococcus aureus*
2. *Streptococcus pyogenes* (Group A)
3. *Neisseria gonorrhoeae*
4. Gram-negative bacilli
5. *Streptococcus pneumoniae*
6. *Neisseria meningitidis*
7. *Haemophilus influenzae* (in children)
8. *Mycobacterium tuberculosis* and other *Mycobacteria*
9. Fungi
10. *Borrelia burgdorferi*

*A protozoan

SKIN AND SUBCUTANEOUS TISSUES

Burns

1. *Staphylococcus aureus*
2. *Streptococcus pyogenes* (Group A)
3. *Pseudomonas aeruginosa* (or other gram-negative bacilli)

Skin infections

1. *Staphylococcus aureus*
2. *Streptococcus pyogenes* (Group A)
3. Dermatophytes
4. *Candida albicans*
5. Herpes simplex or zoster
6. Gram-negative bacilli
7. *Treponema pallidum*
8. *Borrelia burgdorferi*
9. *Bartonella henselae* or *quintana*
10. *Bacillus anthracis*

Decubitus Wound infections

1. *Staphylococcus aureus*
2. *Escherichia coli* (or other gram-negative bacilli)
3. *Streptococcus pyogenes* (Group A)
4. Anaerobic streptococci
5. *Clostridia*
6. *Enterococcus*
7. *Bacteroides*

Traumatic and Surgical Wounds

1. *Staphylococcus aureus*
2. Anaerobic streptococci
3. Gram-negative bacilli
4. *Clostridia*
5. *Streptococcus pyogenes* (Group A)
6. *Enterococcus*

EYES (Cornea and Conjunctiva)

1. Herpes and other viruses
2. *Neisseria gonorrhoeae* (in newborn)
3. *Staphylococcus aureus*
4. *Streptococcus pneumoniae*
5. *Haemophilus influenzae* (in children), including biotype *aegyptius* (Koch-Weeks bacillus)
6. *Moraxella lacunata*
7. *Pseudomonas aeruginosa*
8. Other gram-negative bacilli
9. *Chlamydia trachomatis* (trachoma and inclusion conjunctivitis)
10. Fungi

EARS

Auditory Canal

1. *Pseudomonas aeruginosa* (or other gram-negative bacilli)
2. *Staphylococcus aureus*
3. *Streptococcus pyogenes* (Group A)
4. *Streptococcus pneumoniae*
5. *Haemophilus influenzae* (in children)
6. Fungi

Middle Ear

1. *Streptococcus pneumoniae*
2. *Haemophilus influenzae* (in children)
3. *Moraxella catarrhalis*
4. *Streptococcus pyogenes* (Group A)
5. *Staphylococcus aureus*
6. Anaerobic streptococci (chronic)
7. *Bacteroides* (chronic)
8. Other gram-negative bacilli (chronic)
9. *Mycobacterium tuberculosis*

PARANASAL SINUSES

1. *Streptococcus pneumoniae*
2. *Haemophilus influenzae*
3. *Moraxella catarrhalis*
4. *Streptococcus pyogenes* (Group A)
5. Anaerobic streptococci (chronic sinusitis)
6. *Staphylococcus aureus* (chronic sinusitis)
7. *Klebsiella* (or other gram-negative bacilli)
8. *Mucor, Aspergillus* (especially in diabetics and immunosuppressed patients)

MOUTH

1. Herpes viruses
2. *Candida albicans*
3. *Leptotrichia buccalis* (Vincent's infection)
4. *Bacteroides*
5. Mixed anaerobes
6. *Treponema pallidum*
7. *Actinomyces*

THROAT

1. Respiratory viruses
2. *Streptococcus pyogenes* (Group A)
3. *Neisseria meningitidis* or *gonorrhoeae*
4. *Leptotrichia buccalis*
5. *Candida albicans*
6. *Corynebacterium diphtheriae*
7. *Bordetella pertussis*
8. *Haemophilus influenzae*
9. *Fusobacterium necrophorum*

LARYNX, TRACHEA, AND BRONCHI

1. Respiratory viruses
2. *Streptococcus pneumoniae*
3. *Haemophilus influenzae*
4. *Streptococcus pyogenes* (Group A)
5. *Corynebacterium diphtheriae*
6. *Staphylococcus aureus*
7. Gram-negative bacilli
8. *Fusobacterium necrophorum*

PLEURA

1. *Streptococcus pneumoniae*
2. *Staphylococcus aureus*
3. *Haemophilus influenzae*
4. Gram-negative bacilli
5. Anaerobic streptococci
6. *Bacteroides*
7. *Streptococcus pyogenes* (Group A)
8. *Mycobacterium tuberculosis*
9. *Actinomyces, Nocardia*
10. Fungi
11. *Fusobacterium necrophorum*

LUNGS

Pneumonia

1. Respiratory viruses (influenza virus A and B, adenovirus, respiratory syncytial virus, parainfluenza virus, rhinovirus, enteroviruses, cytomegalovirus, Epstein-Barr virus, varicella-zoster virus, measles virus, herpes simplex virus, hantavirus)
2. *Mycoplasma pneumoniae*
3. *Streptococcus pneumoniae*
4. *Haemophilus influenzae*
5. Anaerobic streptococci, fusospirochetes
6. *Bacteroides*
7. *Staphylococcus aureus*
8. *Klebsiella* (or other gram-negative bacilli)
9. *Legionella pneumophila*
10. *Chlamydia pneumoniae* (TWAR strain)
11. *Streptococcus pyogenes* (Group A)
12. *Rickettsia*
13. *Mycobacterium tuberculosis*
14. *Pneumocystis carinii*
15. Fungi (especially *Aspergillus* species in immunosuppressed patients)
16. *Moraxella catarrhalis*
17. *Legionella micdadei (L. pittsburgensis)*
18. *Chlamydia psittaci*
19. *Fusobacterium necrophorum*
20. *Actinomyces* spp.
21. *Nocardia* spp.
22. *Rhodococcus equi*
23. *Bacillus anthracis*
24. *Yersinia pestis*

Abscess

1. Anaerobic streptococci
2. *Bacteroides*
3. *Staphylococcus aureus*
4. *Klebsiella* (or other gram-negative bacilli)
5. *Streptococcus pneumoniae*
6. Fungi
7. *Actinomyces, Nocardia*

GASTROINTESTINAL TRACT

1. Gastrointestinal viruses
2. *Campylobacter jejuni*
3. *Salmonella*
4. *Escherichia coli*
5. *Shigella*
6. *Yersinia enterocolitica*
7. *Entamoeba histolytica**
8. *Giardia lamblia**
9. *Staphylococcus aureus*
10. *Vibrio cholerae*
11. *Vibrio parahaemolyticus*
12. Herpes simplex (anus)
13. *Treponema pallidum* (rectum)
14. *Neisseria gonorrhoeae* (rectum)
15. *Candida albicans*
16. *Clostridium difficile*
17. *Cryptosporidium parvum**
18. Cytomegalovirus
19. Human immunodeficiency virus (HIV)
20. *Mycobacterium avium* complex
21. *Helicobacter pylori*
22. *Tropheryma whippelii*

*A protozoan

URINARY TRACT

1. *Escherichia coli* (or other gram-negative bacilli)
2. *Staphylococcus aureus* and *epidermidis*
3. *Neisseria gonorrhoeae* (urethra)
4. *Enterococcus*
5. *Candida albicans*
6. *Chlamydia* (urethra)
7. *Treponema pallidum* (urethra)
8. *Trichomonas vaginalis** (urethra)
9. *Ureaplasma urealyticum*

FEMALE GENITAL TRACT

Vagina

1. *Trichomonas vaginalis**
2. *Candida albicans*
3. *Neisseria gonorrhoeae*
4. *Streptococcus pyogenes* (Group A)
5. *Gardnerella vaginalis* and associated anaerobes
6. *Treponema pallidum*

Uterus

1. Anaerobic streptococci
2. *Bacteroides*
3. *Neisseria gonorrhoeae* (cervix)
4. *Clostridia*
5. *Escherichia coli* (or other gram-negative bacilli)
6. Herpes virus, type II (cervix)
7. *Streptococcus pyogenes* (Group A)
8. *Streptococcus*, Groups B and C
9. *Treponema pallidum*
10. *Actinomyces* spp. (most common infection of intrauterine devices)
11. *Staphylococcus aureus*
11. *Enterococcus*
12. *Chlamydia trachomatis*
13. *Mycoplasma hominis*

Fallopian Tubes

1. *Neisseria gonorrhoeae*
2. *Escherichia coli* (or other gram-negative bacilli)
3. Anaerobic streptococci
4. *Bacteroides*
5. *Chlamydia trachomatis*

MALE GENITAL TRACT

Seminal Vesicles

1. Gram-negative bacilli
2. *Neisseria gonorrhoeae*

Epididymis

1. *Chlamydia*
2. Gram-negative bacilli
3. *Neisseria gonorrhoeae*
4. *Mycobacterium tuberculosis*

Prostate Gland

1. Gram-negative bacilli
2. *Neisseria gonorrhoeae*

PERITONEUM

1. Gram-negative bacilli
2. *Enterococcus*
3. *Bacteroides*
4. Anaerobic streptococci
5. *Clostridia*
6. *Streptococcus pneumoniae*
7. *Streptococcus* Group B

*A protozoan

ANTIMICROBIAL SUSCEPTIBILITY TESTS

Most clinical laboratories test bacterial isolates for susceptibility to antimicrobial drugs with a disk diffusion test or semi- or fully-automated methods that find the minimum inhibitory concentrations (MICs) of different antibiotics for each isolate and convert those data to designations of "susceptible," "intermediate" (sometimes called "indeterminate") or "resistant." All of these methods are designed to test the susceptibility of common bacterial pathogens such as staphylococci and rapidly growing aerobic gram-negative rods. Modified methods have been developed for testing the antimicrobial susceptibility of certain organisms that have recently developed antibiotic resistance, particularly *Streptococcus pneumoniae* and *Enterococcus*.

THE DISK DIFFUSION TEST — A suspension of the bacterial strain is swabbed on Mueller-Hinton agar, and 10 to 12 antimicrobial disks are placed on the surface of a 150-mm plate. After incubation for about 18 hours (overnight), the diameter of the zone of growth inhibition around each disk indicates whether the isolate is "resistant," "intermediate" or "susceptible;" these characterizations are based on a correlation of the zone sizes and results of quantitative dilution tests obtained with each drug against many different bacterial strains, and on the usual plasma concentrations of the drug obtained with recommended doses.

OTHER TESTS OF SUSCEPTIBILITY — Dilution susceptibility tests use various concentrations of the antibiotic in Mueller-Hinton broth or in agar, which are then inoculated with a standardized concentration of the test organism and incubated for about 18 hours. The MIC of the antibiotic is the lowest drug concentration that inhibits growth, as detected by the absence of turbidity in the tube or of visible growth on the plate. The E-test (epsilometer test) is performed with a strip containing a gradient of the antibiotic to be tested; the strip is placed on an inoculated plate and zone size is read as the MIC (JH Jorgensen and MJ Ferraro, Clin Infect Dis

1998; 26:973). Other tests of susceptibility use automated equipment that determines in only a few hours how an antibiotic changes the turbidity or other characteristics of a growing bacterial culture; then a computer program converts these data to the MIC of the antibiotic and determines whether the isolate is "susceptible," "intermediate" or "resistant."

LIMITATIONS OF SUSCEPTIBILITY TESTS — Differences in Dosage – The designations of "susceptible," "intermediate" and "resistant" are based on average serum concentrations obtained with the usual doses of a particular drug, but many different dosage schedules are used, and antimicrobial serum concentrations vary even among patients on the same dosage schedule.

Site of Infection – Antibiotic concentrations in cerebrospinal fluid are more important than serum concentrations in meningitis. In endocarditis or meningitis, broth or agar dilution tests that give quantitative results (MIC and minimum bactericidal concentration [MBC]) may be preferred over disk tests, which indicate inhibition of growth but not necessarily bactericidal activity. With most antimicrobial drugs, the concentration in urine is much higher than in blood; therefore, an antimicrobial may sometimes be effective for treating a urinary tract infection even when a disk test based on achievable plasma concentrations is read as "intermediate" or "resistant." With sulfonamides, nitrofurantoin, nalidixic acid, cinoxacin and trimethoprim, usual urinary concentrations are used as the basis for interpretation of disk tests.

Organisms – The standard disk-diffusion test is not usually recommended for ***Haemophilus influenzae*** (for testing susceptibility to ampicillin or amoxicillin), **meningococci, gonococci, tubercle bacilli** or ***Nocardia***, which should be tested by other methods. ***H. influenzae*** should be tested for β-lactamase production (to test susceptibility to ampicillin or amoxicillin) as soon as the culture grows, followed by the E-test or a disk diffusion or dilution test for susceptibility to other antimicrobial agents. Some isolates of *H. influenzae* will be β-lactamase negative on screening, but positive when tested by disk diffusion or other standard methods. Isolates of ***Neisseria gonorrhoeae*** should also be tested for β-lactamase production, but some relatively penicillin-resistant strains may not produce β-lactamase. Special standardized disk diffusion susceptibility tests for gonococci have been described (National Committee for Clinical Laboratory Standards, *Performance Standards for Antimicrobial Disk Susceptibility Tests*, 7th ed., Approved Standard [M2-A7 - Supplement M100-S11], Wayne, PA:NCCLS, 2002). Some gram-negative bacilli produce extended-spectrum β-lactamases that inactivate penicillins, cephalosporins and aztreonam, but the resistance may be difficult to detect by routine methods such as disk diffusion. Ceftazidime is highly susceptible to such inactivation; a ceftazidime disk, sometimes combined with a disk containing a β-lactamase inhibitor, can be used to screen for this type of resistance.

Currently, no procedure is universally accepted for testing antimicrobial susceptibility of **anaerobes**, but some guidelines have been proposed (National Committee for Clinical Laboratory Standards, *Methods for Antimicrobial Susceptibility Testing of Anaerobic Bacteria*, 5th ed., Approved Standard [M11-A5], Wayne, PA:NCCLS, 2000). The E-test compares well with agar dilution tests for some faster growing anaerobes such as *Bacteroides*.

With **enterococci**, ordinary disk susceptibility tests are often misleading; enterococcal endocarditis or other intravascular infections require either a penicillin or vancomycin plus an aminoglycoside for adequate therapy, even if the organisms are susceptible to one drug *in vitro*. Special attention needs to be directed to detection of susceptibility of enterococci to vancomycin and to ampicillin; the E-test can be helpful (JE Schulz and DF Sahm, J Clin Microbiol 1993; 31:3336). Susceptibility of enterococci to aminoglycosides is determined by special agar plate or tube dilution sensitivity tests. The latter are used to determine whether adding an aminoglycoside to either a β-lactam or vancomycin would have a synergistic effect. Strains of ***S. pneumoniae*** **(pneumococci)** may be resistant to penicillin; isolates should be screened for penicillin susceptibility using an oxacillin disk test. If resistance is detected to penicillin, the degree of resistance to penicillin and susceptibility to other antimicrobial agents is determined by a dilution test or the E-test.

Antimicrobial Agents – Strains of *Staphylococcus aureus* and coagulase-negative staphylococci resistant to one of the **penicillinase-resistant penicillins** (often called "methicillin-resistant" strains) are generally resistant to the others and also to the cephalosporins, regardless of *in vitro* results with cephalosporin disks, and to other β-lactams such as imipenem. Use of oxacillin disks (rather than methicillin or nafcillin), and incubation at 35°C (rather than 37°C) for 24 hours improves detection of methicillin resistance. In addition, special dilution susceptibility tests are sometimes used to detect methicillin-resistant staphylococci. The most reliable of these is the oxacillin agar plate. Testing the sulfonamide susceptibility of fastidious organisms such as meningococci requires specialized techniques; routine tests can result in erroneous reports of either susceptibility or resistance. Results of susceptibility tests with **tetracycline** are usually applicable to all tetracyclines. Staphylococci, *Nocardia*, and some nonfermenters such as *Acinetobacter*, however, are sometimes more susceptible to doxycycline and minocycline than to tetracycline. Cephalothin is the recommended routine disk for most first-generation **cephalosporins** (cefadroxil, cephalexin, cephapirin, and cephradine) and also for cefaclor. Cefazolin, also a first-generation cephalosporin, is more active against *Escherichia coli* and has its own disk. There is no true class disk for either the second-generation cephalosporins (cefoxitin, cefonicid, cefamandole, cefotetan, cefmetazole, cefpodoxime, cefprozil, cefuroxime and loracarbef), the third-generation cephalosporins (cefotaxime, cefoperazone, ceftizoxime, ceftriaxone, ceftazidime, cefixime, cefditoren and ceftibuten) or the fourth-generation cephalosporin cefepime. Susceptibility to third-generation cephalosporins does not predict susceptibility to fourth-generation cephalosporins. Unlike other cephalosporins, cefixime and ceftibuten (Medical Letter 1996; 38:23) are not active against staphylococci.

WHICH ANTIMICROBIALS TO TEST — The recent approval of many new antimicrobial drugs has created a problem for clinical bacteriology laboratories using disk diffusion susceptibility tests because antibiotic disk plates have places for a maximum of 12 disks and trays of antibiotics used for automated dilution systems are prepackaged by the manufacturers. Few laboratories using the disk method have the financial resources to inoculate two plates to test more than 12 antibiotics routinely, or to purchase customized trays of antibiotics for use in the automated system. Some examples of disks that might be appropriate for routine testing in a laboratory that serves both inpatients and outpatients are listed in the table on page 32. These choices reflect suggestions of Medical Letter consultants, but not unanimity, and local patterns of bacterial resistance and antimicrobial usage would undoubtedly dictate some changes. Some laboratories withhold information on newer, more expensive drugs when organisms are susceptible to less expensive agents.

CONCLUSION — Standardized susceptibility tests can help guide the choice of an antimicrobial agent, but the patient's response to adequate doses of an antimicrobial drug is the ultimate test of its usefulness against the infecting organism. A poor response to a drug used against a "susceptible" organism may indicate that the drug is not reaching the organism, or that either surgical drainage or larger doses are required.

SOME DISKS FOR ROUTINE TESTING

Gram-Negative Isolates[1] (except *Pseudomonas*) From Urine[2]	Gram-Negative Isolates[1] (except *Pseudomonas*) From Other Sites[3]	Gram-Positive Isolate[4,5]	*Pseudomonas*[1]
amikacin[6]	amikacin[6]	amikacin[6, 14]	amikacin[6]
amoxicillin/clavulanic acid	ampicillin[7]	amoxicillin/clavulanic acid	aztreonam
ampicillin[7]	cefotaxime, ceftizoxime or ceftriaxone[11]	cephalothin[7]	carbenicillin[16]
cefotaxime, ceftizoxime or ceftriaxone[11]	cefoxitin or cefotetan	clindamycin	cefepime
cephalothin[7]	ceftazidime	erythromycin	ceftazidime
ciprofloxacin[8]	cephalothin[7]	gentamicin[14]	ciprofloxacin[8]
gentamicin[9]	ciprofloxacin[8]	levofloxacin[15]	gentamicin[9]
nitrofurantoin	gentamicin[9]	oxacillin[7]	imipenem[12]
piperacillin[10]	imipenem[12]	penicillin	piperacillin or ticarcillin
sulfisoxazole[7]	piperacillin/tazobactam[13]	trimethoprim/sulfamethoxazole	tobramycin
tetracycline[7]	piperacillin[10]	vancomycin	trimethoprim/sulfamethoxazole[17]
trimethoprim/sulfamethoxazole	trimethoprim/sulfamethoxazole		

1. Susceptibility of gram-negative organisms may vary widely from hospital to hospital and modifications may be appropriate.
2. If more than 12 antibiotics can be tested, some institutions add cefixime, fosfomycin, cefepime, ceftazidime and aztreonam.
3. If more than 12 antibiotics can be tested, some institutions add cefepime and aztreonam.
4. Enterococci should not be tested by the disk-diffusion method because the results are often misleading. For enterococci isolated from normally sterile body fluids or other clinically relevant cultures, most laboratories use an E-test or tube dilution to test susceptibility to ampicillin, vancomycin, ciprofloxacin, chloramphenicol, trimethoprim/sulfamethoxazole, doxycycline and quinupristin/dalfopristin *(Synercid)*. Susceptibility of enterococci to aminoglycosides is determined by special agar plate or tube dilution sensitivity tests.
5. For *S. pneumoniae*, most laboratories use oxacillin disk screening for penicillin susceptibility. If screening suggests either intermediate or high-level resistance, a tube dilution or E-test can be used to test susceptibility to penicillin, vancomycin, erythromycin, trimethoprim/sulfamethoxazole, cefotaxime, ceftriaxone, azithromycin, clarithromycin, and either levofloxacin, gatifloxacin or moxifloxacin.

6. Some laboratories do not report amikacin unless organism is resistant to gentamicin.
7. Represents the class disk for some related antimicrobials; one of these could be substituted.
8. Or levofloxacin, gatifloxacin or moxifloxacin.
9. Tobramycin is similar but is more active *in vitro* against some strains of *Pseudomonas.*
10. Or ticarcillin. Some gram-negative strains resistant to ticarcillin may be susceptible to piperacillin.
11. Non-pseudomonas gram-negative isolates susceptible to these drugs are usually also susceptible to aztreonam and ceftazidime.
12. Or meropenem.
13. Ticarcillin/clavulanic acid may be substituted.
14. Should not be used alone; sometimes combined with a penicillin or a cephalosporin to treat staphylococcal infections.
15. Or gatifloxacin or moxifloxacin.
16. To predict susceptibility to indanyl carbenicillin for oral use.
17. *Pseudomonas aeruginosa* strains are resistant, but other *Pseudomonas* species are sometimes susceptible.

THE CHOICE OF ANTIBACTERIAL DRUGS

New drugs for bacterial infections and new information about older drugs continue to become available. Empirical treatment of some infections is discussed below. A table listing the drugs of choice and alternatives for each pathogen begins on page 40. These recommendations are based on results of susceptibility studies, clinical trials and the opinions of Medical Letter consultants. Local resistance patterns should be taken into account.

PNEUMONIA — Community-acquired bacterial pneumonia is frequently caused by *Streptococcus pneumoniae* (pneumococci). In the United States, more than 15% of recent isolates of *S. pneumoniae* are highly resistant to penicillin and increasingly resistant to cephalosporins, macrolides, and less commonly to fluoroquinolones. Other bacterial pathogens include *Haemophilus influenzae, Staphylococcus aureus, Klebsiella pneumoniae* and occasionally other gram-negative bacilli and anaerobic mouth organisms. "Atypical" pathogens, including *Mycoplasma pneumoniae, Chlamydia pneumoniae* and respiratory viruses are probably the most common cause of community-acquired pneumonia. *Legionella,* another "atypical" organism, is less common. Tuberculosis, *Pneumocystis carinii* pneumonia and regionally endemic fungal infections, such as histoplasmosis or coccidioidomycosis, must also be considered in the differential diagnosis (JG Bartlett et al, Clin Infect Dis 2000; 31:347).

In patients who require hospitalization, cefotaxime or ceftriaxone is a reasonable first choice pending culture results, antibiotic susceptibility testing and clinical response. To cover *Legionella, Mycoplasma* and *Chlamydia,* a macrolide (erythromycin, azithromycin or clarithromycin) is often added, or a fluoroquinolone with good activity against *S. pneumoniae* (such as levofloxacin, gatifloxacin or moxifloxacin) can be substituted for both the β-lactam and the macrolide. When aspiration pneumonia is suspected, metronidazole or clindamycin can be added. In treating pneumococcal pneumonia due to strains with intermediate degrees of penicillin resistance (minimal inhibitory concentration [MIC] 0.1 to <2 μg/ml), cefotaxime, ceftriaxone or high doses of intravenous (IV) penicillin (12 million units daily for adults) can be used. For highly resistant strains (MIC ≥ 2 μg/ml), an IV fluoroquinolone (levofloxacin, gatifloxacin or moxifloxacin) or vancomycin may be required, and should be added in all severely ill patients and those not responding to a β-lactam.

In ambulatory patients, an oral macrolide, doxycycline or a fluoroquinolone with good anti-pneumococcal activity (such as levofloxacin, gatifloxacin or moxifloxacin) is recommended for otherwise healthy adults. Pneumococci may, however, be resistant to a macrolide or doxycycline, especially if they are resistant to penicillin; for older patients or those with underlying disease, a fluoroquinolone may be a better choice.

Hospital-acquired bacterial pneumonia is often caused by gram-negative bacilli, especially *Klebsiella, Enterobacter, Serratia, Acinetobacter* and *Pseudomonas aeruginosa*, as well as *Staphylococcus aureus*. Antimicrobial resistance is frequent in these organisms and can emerge during treatment. For initial treatment Medical Letter consultants would use an aminoglycoside (tobramycin, gentamicin or amikacin) plus one of the following: cefotaxime, ceftriaxone, cefepime, ticarcillin/clavulanic acid, piperacillin/tazobactam, meropenem or imipenem. The third-generation cephalosporins cefotaxime, ceftizoxime and ceftriaxone have poor activity against *Pseudomonas*. Ceftazidime has good activity against *Pseudomonas* but poor activity against staphylococci, other gram-positive cocci and anaerobes. In intensive care units where *Pseudomonas aeruginosa* and other highly-resistant gram-negative organisms are frequently the cause of nosocomial pneumonia, cefepime, imipenem, or meropenem combined with an aminoglycoside would be a good first choice. Addition of vancomycin should be considered in hospitals where methicillin-resistant staphylococci are prevalent.

MENINGITIS — The organisms most commonly responsible for community-acquired bacterial meningitis are *S. pneumoniae* and *Neisseria meningitidis*. Meningitis due to *H. influenzae* type b in children has decreased markedly as a result of immunization. Enteric gram-negative bacteria cause meningitis especially in newborn infants, patients more than 60 years old, and in those who have had neurosurgery or are immunosuppressed. Group B streptococcus may cause meningitis in neonates. *Listeria monocytogenes* may also be the cause in pregnant women and newborns and in the elderly or immunosuppressed.

For treatment of meningitis in adults and in children more than two months old, pending results of cultures, high-dose cefotaxime or ceftriaxone is generally recommended, plus vancomycin with or without rifampin to cover resistant pneumococci. Vancomycin in usual doses may not reach effective levels in cerebrospinal fluid; some Medical Letter consultants have used 4 grams per day to treat meningitis. Both vancomycin and rifampin should be stopped if the etiologic agent proves to be susceptible to cephalosporins. For treatment of nosocomial meningitis, vancomycin and a cephalosporin with good activity against *Pseudomonas* such as ceftazidime are appropriate; if *Pseudomonas* is confirmed, addition of an aminoglycoside (tobramycin, gentamicin or amikacin) is recommended. Meningitis due to *Listeria* should be treated with ampicillin, with or without gentamicin.

In Penicillin-Allergic Patients – Cefotaxime or ceftriaxone is sometimes used to treat meningitis in penicillin-allergic patients, but such patients may also have allergic reactions to cephalosporins. Vancomycin with or without rifampin should be added to cover resistant pneumococci. When allergy prevents the use of a cephalosporin, chloramphenicol can be given for initial treatment, but may not be effective if the pathogens are enteric gram-negative bacilli or *Listeria*, or in some patients with pneumococcal meningitis. For enteric gram-negative bacilli, aztreonam could be used. Trimethoprim-sulfamethoxazole can be used for treatment of *Listeria* meningitis in patients allergic to penicillin.

Use of Corticosteroids – Whether dexamethasone (*Decadron*, and others) given before or at the same time as the first dose of antibiotics decreases the incidence of hearing loss and other neurological complications in children with meningitis remains controversial (PK Coyle, Arch Neurol 1999; 56:796).

In Newborns – Neonatal meningitis is most often caused by group B or other streptococci, gram-negative enteric organisms or *Listeria*. For meningitis in the first two months of life, while waiting for the results of cultures and susceptibility tests, many Medical Letter consultants use ampicillin plus cefotaxime, with or without gentamicin.

SEPSIS SYNDROME — For treatment of a sepsis syndrome, the choice of drugs should be based on the probable source of infection, gram-stained smears of appropriate clinical specimens and the immune status of the patient. The choice should also reflect local patterns of bacterial resistance.

A third- or fourth-generation cephalosporin (cefotaxime, ceftizoxime, ceftriaxone, cefepime or ceftazidime), imipenem or meropenem, or aztreonam can be used to treat sepsis caused by many strains of gram-negative bacilli. Ceftazidime has less activity against gram-positive cocci. Cephalosporins other than ceftazidime and cefepime have limited activity against *Pseudomonas aeruginosa*. Imipenem, meropenem and aztreonam are active against most strains of *P. aeruginosa*, and imipenem and meropenem are active against anaerobes. Aztreonam has no activity against gram-positive bacteria or anaerobes.

Initial Treatment – For initial treatment of life-threatening sepsis in adults, Medical Letter consultants recommend either a third- or fourth-generation cephalosporin (cefotaxime, ceftriaxone or cefepime), ticarcillin/clavulanic acid, piperacillin/tazobactam, imipenem or meropenem, each together with an aminoglycoside (gentamicin, tobramycin or amikacin). When methicillin-resistant staphylococci are suspected, treatment with vancomycin (alone or with gentamicin and/or rifampin) is often recommended. When bacterial endocarditis is suspected and therapy must be started before the pathogen is identified, a combination of vancomycin and gentamicin can be used.

For intra-abdominal or pelvic infections likely to involve anaerobes, treatment should include either ticarcillin/clavulanic acid, ampicillin/sulbactam, piperacillin/tazobactam, cefoxitin or cefotetan or a carbapenem such as imipenem, each with or without an aminoglycoside. When the source of bacteremia is thought to be in the biliary tract, some clinicians would use piperacillin plus metronidazole, piperacillin/tazobactam or ampicillin/sulbactam, each with or without an aminoglycoside.

Neutropenic Patients – For suspected bacteremia in neutropenic patients, ceftazidime, imipenem, meropenem or cefepime, each alone or in more seriously ill patients with an aminoglycoside (gentamicin, tobramycin or amikacin), would be a reasonable first choice. Piperacillin/tazobactam (4.5 grams q6h) or ticarcillin/clavulanic acid (3.1 gram q4h), either combined with amikacin, may be equally effective. Addition of vancomycin may be necessary for treatment of neutropenic patients who remain febrile despite antibiotics or who develop bacteremia caused by methicillin-resistant staphylococci or penicillin-resistant viridans streptococci.

Studies in low-risk hospitalized adults show that when neutropenia is expected to last less than 10 days, oral ciprofloxacin with amoxicillin/clavulanic acid is as effective as intravenous ceftazidime or ceftriaxone plus amikacin (A Freifeld et al, N Engl J Med 1999; 341:305; WV Kern et al, N Engl J Med 1999; 341:312).

Antibiotic-Resistant Gram-Negative Bacilli – In some hospitals, gram-negative bacilli have become increasingly resistant to aminoglycosides, third-generation cephalosporins and aztreonam; these strains may be susceptible to imipenem, meropenem, ertapenem, ciprofloxacin or trimethoprim-sulfamethoxazole. Resistance is also increasing in some community-acquired organisms such as *Salmonella* spp. and *Shigella* spp. (EF Dunne et al, JAMA 2000; 284:3151; RL Shapiro et al, J Infect Dis 2001; 183:1701). Susceptibility testing and resistance patterns within the region, as reported by public health laboratories, should be used to guide therapy.

Multiple-antibiotic-resistant enterococci – Many *Enterococcus* spp. are now resistant to penicillin and ampicillin, gentamicin or streptomycin or both, and to vancomycin. Some of these strains are susceptible *in vitro* to chloramphenicol, doxycycline or fluoroquinolones, but clinical results with these drugs have been variable. Linezolid (Medical Letter 2000; 42:45), an oxazolidinone, is active against many gram-positive organisms, including both *Enterococcus faecium* and *Enterococcus faecalis* (JW Chien et al, Clin Infect Dis 2000; 30:146). Quinupristin/dalfopristin (Medical Letter 1999; 41:109) is active against most strains of vancomycin-resistant *E. faecium*, but not *E. faecalis* (DJ Winston et al, Clin Infect Dis 2000; 30:790). Polymicrobial surgical infections that include antibiotic-resistant enterococci may respond to antibiotics aimed at the other organisms. When antibiotic-resistant enterococci cause endocarditis, surgical replacement of the infected valve may be required. Urinary tract infections caused by resistant enterococci may respond nevertheless to ampicillin or amoxicillin, which reach very high concentrations in urine; nitrofurantoin or fosfomycin can also be used.

URINARY TRACT INFECTION — Acute uncomplicated cystitis in women can be effectively and inexpensively treated, before the infecting organism is known, with a three-day course of oral trimethoprim-sulfamethoxazole; in areas where the prevalence of *E. coli* resistant to trimethoprim-sulfamethoxazole exceeds 15% to 20%, a fluoroquinolone can be substituted (JW Warren, Clin Infect Dis 1999; 29:745; K Gupta et al, Ann Intern Med 2001; 135:41). Other alternatives include five- to seven-day regimens of nitrofurantoin, an oral cephalosporin, or a single dose of fosfomycin. Acute uncomplicated pyelonephritis can often be managed with a seven-day course of an oral fluoroquinolone (DA Talan et al, JAMA 2000; 283:1583). Urinary tract infections that recur after use of antimicrobial agents or are acquired in hospitals or nursing homes are more likely to be due to antibiotic-resistant gram-negative bacilli, *S. aureus* or enterococci. A fluoroquinolone, oral amoxicillin/clavulanic acid or an oral third-generation cephalosporin (cefixime, cefpodoxime, cefdinir or ceftibuten) can be useful in treating such infections in outpatients. In hospitalized patients with urinary tract infections, treatment with a third-generation cephalosporin, a fluoroquinolone, ticarcillin/clavulanic acid, piperacillin/tazobactam, imipenem or meropenem is recommended, sometimes together with an aminoglycoside, such as gentamicin, especially in patients with a sepsis syndrome.

ANTIBACTERIAL DRUGS OF CHOICE

Infecting Organism	Drug of First Choice	Alternative Drugs
GRAM-POSITIVE COCCI		
**Enterococcus*[1]		
endocarditis or other severe infection	penicillin G or ampicillin + gentamicin or streptomycin[2]	vancomycin + gentamicin or streptomycin[2]; linezolid; quinupristin/dalfopristin
uncomplicated urinary tract infection	ampicillin or amoxicillin	nitrofurantoin; a fluoroquinolone[3]; fosfomycin
**Staphylococcus aureus* or *epidermidis*		
methicillin-sensitive	a penicillinase-resistant penicillin[4]	a cephalosporin[5,6]; vancomycin; amoxicillin/clavulanic acid; ticarcillin/clavulanic acid; piperacillin/tazobactam; ampicillin/sulbactam; imipenem or meropenem; clindamycin; a fluoroquinolone[3]
methicillin-resistant[7]	vancomycin ± gentamicin ± rifampin	linezolid; quinupristin/dalfopristin; a fluoroquinolone[3]; a tetracycline[8]; trimethoprim-sulfamethoxazole

* **Resistance may be a problem; susceptibility tests should be used to guide therapy.**

1. Disk sensitivity testing may not provide adequate information; β-lactamase assays, "E" tests and dilution tests for susceptibility should be used in serious infections.
2. Aminoglycoside resistance is increasingly common among enterococci; treatment options include ampicillin 2 g IV q4h, continuous infusion of ampicillin, a combination of ampicillin plus a fluoroquinolone, or a combination of ampicillin, imipenem and vancomycin.
3. Among the fluoroquinolones, levofloxacin, gatifloxacin and moxifloxacin have excellent *in vitro* activity against *S. pneumoniae,* including penicillin- and cephalosporin-resistant strains. Levofloxacin, gatifloxacin and moxifloxacin also have good activity against many strains of *S. aureus,* but resistance has become frequent among methicillin-resistant strains. Ciprofloxacin has the greatest activity against *Pseudomonas aeruginosa.* For urinary tract infections, norfloxacin, lomefloxacin or enoxacin can be used. For tuberculosis, levofloxacin, ofloxacin, ciprofloxacin, gatifloxacin or moxifloxacin could be used. Ciprofloxacin, ofloxacin, levofloxacin, moxifloxacin and gatifloxacin are available for IV use. None of these agents are recommended for children or pregnant women.
4. For oral use against staphylococci, cloxacillin or dicloxacillin is preferred; for severe infections, a parenteral formulation of nafcillin or oxacillin should be used. Ampicillin, amoxicillin, carbenicillin, ticarcillin and piperacillin are not effective against penicillinase-producing staphylococci. The combinations of clavulanic acid with amoxicillin or ticarcillin, sulbactam with ampicillin, and tazobactam with piperacillin may be active against these organisms.

Infecting Organism	Drug of First Choice	Alternative Drugs
Streptococcus pyogenes (group A[9]) and groups C and G	penicillin G or V[10]	clindamycin; erythromycin; a cephalosporin[5,6]; vancomycin; clarithromycin[11]; azithromycin

5. The cephalosporins have been used as alternatives to penicillins in patients allergic to penicillins, but such patients may also have allergic reactions to cephalosporins.
6. For parenteral treatment of staphylococcal or non-enterococcal streptococcal infections, a first-generation cephalosporin such as cefazolin can be used. For oral therapy, cephalexin or cephradine can be used. The second-generation cephalosporins cefamandole, cefprozil, cefuroxime, cefonicid, cefotetan, cefoxitin and loracarbef are more active than the first-generation drugs against gram-negative bacteria. Cefuroxime is active against ampicillin-resistant strains of *H. influenzae.* Cefoxitin and cefotetan are the most active of the cephalosporins against *B. fragilis,* but cefotetan has been associated with prothrombin deficiency. The third-generation cephalosporins cefotaxime, cefoperazone, ceftizoxime, ceftriaxone and ceftazidime and the "fourth-generation" cefepime have greater activity than the second-generation drugs against enteric gram-negative bacilli. Ceftazidime has poor activity against many gram-positive cocci and anaerobes, and ceftizoxime has poor activity against penicillin-resistant *S. pneumoniae.* Cefepime has *in vitro* activity against gram-positive cocci similar to cefotaxime and ceftriaxone and somewhat greater activity against enteric gram-negative bacilli. The activity of cefepime against *Pseudomonas aeruginosa* is similar to that of ceftazidime. Cefixime, cefpodoxime, cefdinir, ceftibuten and cefditoren are oral cephalosporins with more activity than second-generation cephalosporins against facultative gram-negative bacilli; they have no useful activity against anaerobes or *P. aeruginosa,* and cefixime and ceftibuten have no useful activity against staphylococci. With the exception of cefoperazone (which, like cefamandole, can cause bleeding), ceftazidime and cefepime, the activity of all currently available cephalosporins against *P. aeruginosa* is poor or inconsistent.
7. Many strains of coagulase-positive staphylococci and coagulase-negative staphylococci are resistant to penicillinase-resistant penicillins; these strains are also resistant to cephalosporins, imipenem and meropenem, and are often resistant to fluoroquinolones, trimethoprim/sulfamethoxazole and clindamycin.
8. Tetracyclines are generally not recommended for pregnant women or children less than 8 years old.
9. For serious soft-tissue infection due to group A streptococci, clindamycin may be more effective than penicillin. Group A streptococci may, however, be resistant to clindamycin; therefore, some Medical Letter consultants suggest using both clindamycin and penicillin, with or without IV immune globulin, to treat serious soft-tissue infections. Group A streptococci may also be resistant to erythromycin, azithromycin and clarithromycin.
10. Penicillin V (or amoxicillin) is preferred for oral treatment of infections caused by non-penicillinase-producing streptococci. For initial therapy of severe infections, penicillin G, administered parenterally, is first choice. For somewhat longer action in less severe infections due to group A streptococci, pneumococci or *Treponema pallidum,* procaine penicillin G, an IM formulation, can be given once or twice daily, but is seldom used now. Benzathine penicillin G, a slowly absorbed preparation, is usually given in a single monthly injection for prophylaxis of rheumatic fever, once for treatment of Group A streptococcal pharyngitis and once or more for treatment of syphilis.
11. Not recommended for use in pregnancy.

Infecting Organism	Drug of First Choice	Alternative Drugs
Gram-Positive Cocci *(continued)*		
Streptococcus, group B	penicillin G or ampicillin	a cephalosporin[5,6]; vancomycin; erythromycin
**Streptococcus*, viridans group[1]	penicillin G ± gentamicin	a cephalosporin[5,6]; vancomycin
Streptococcus bovis	penicillin G	a cephalosporin[5,6]; vancomycin
Streptococcus, anaerobic or *Peptostreptococcus*	penicillin G	clindamycin; a cephalosporin[5,6]; vancomycin
**Streptococcus pneumoniae*[12] (pneumococcus), penicillin-susceptible (MIC <0.1 μg/ml)	penicillin G or V[10]; amoxicillin	a cephalosporin[5,6]; erythromycin; azithromycin; clarithromycin[11]; levofloxacin[13], gatifloxacin[13] or moxifloxacin[13]; meropenem; imipenem; ertapenem; trimethoprim-sulfamethoxazole; clindamycin; a tetracycline[8]
penicillin-intermediate resistance (MIC 0.1 - ≤2 μg/ml)	penicillin G IV (12 million units/day for adults); ceftriaxone or cefotaxime	levofloxacin[13], gatifloxacin[13] or moxifloxacin[13]; vancomycin; clindamycin
penicillin-high level resistance (MIC ≥ 2 μg/ml)	**meningitis:** vancomycin + ceftriaxone or cefotaxime, ± rifampin	meropenem
	other infections: vancomycin + ceftriaxone or cefotaxime; or levofloxacin[13], gatifloxacin[13] or moxifloxacin[13]	linezolid; quinupristin/dalfopristin

12. Some strains of *S. pneumoniae* are resistant to erythromycin, clindamycin, trimethoprim-sulfamethoxazole, clarithromycin, azithromycin and chloramphenicol, and resistance to the newer fluoroquinolones is increasing (R Davidson et al, N Engl J Med 2002; 346:747). Nearly all strains tested so far are susceptible to linezolid and quinupristin/dalfopristin *in vitro* (R Patel et al, Diagn Microbiol Infect Dis 1999; 34:119; J Verhaegen and L Verbist, J Antimicrob Chemother 1999; 43:563).
13. Usually not recommended for use in children or pregnant women.

Infecting Organism	Drug of First Choice	Alternative Drugs
GRAM-NEGATIVE COCCI		
Moraxella (Branhamella) catarrhalis	cefuroxime[5]; a fluoroquinolone[3]	trimethoprim-sulfamethoxazole; amoxicillin/clavulanic acid; erythromycin; a tetracycline[8]; cefotaxime[5]; ceftizoxime[5]; ceftriaxone[5]; cefuroxime axetil[5]; cefixime[5]; cefpodoxime[5]; clarithromycin[11]; azithromycin
**Neisseria gonorrhoeae* (gonococcus)[14]	ceftriaxone[5] or cefixime[5]; or ciprofloxacin[13], gatifloxacin[13] or ofloxacin[13]	cefotaxime[5]; penicillin G
Neisseria meningitidis[15] (meningococcus)	penicillin G	cefotaxime[5]; ceftizoxime[5]; ceftriaxone[5]; chloramphenicol[16]; a sulfonamide[17]; a fluoroquinolone[3]
GRAM-POSITIVE BACILLI		
Bacillus anthracis (anthrax)	ciprofloxacin[13]; a tetracycline[8]	penicillin G; erythromycin
Bacillus cereus, subtilis	vancomycin	imipenem or meropenem; clindamycin
Clostridium perfringens[18]	penicillin G; clindamycin	metronidazole; imipenem; meropenem; ertapenem; chloramphenicol[16]
Clostridium tetani[19]	metronidazole	penicillin G; a tetracycline[8]
Clostridium difficile[20]	metronidazole	vancomycin (oral)

14. Patients with gonorrhea should be treated presumptively for co-infection with *C. trachomatis* with azithromycin or doxycycline.
15. Rare strains of *N. meningitidis* are resistant or relatively resistant to penicillin. A fluoroquinolone or rifampin is recommended for prophylaxis after close contact with infected patients.
16. Because of the possibility of serious adverse effects, this drug should be used only for severe infections when less hazardous drugs are ineffective.
17. Sulfonamide-resistant strains are frequent in the US; sulfonamides should be used only when susceptibility is established by susceptibility tests.
18. Debridement is primary. Large doses of penicillin G are required. Hyperbaric oxygen therapy may be a useful adjunct to surgical debridement in management of the spreading, necrotizing type of infection.
19. For prophylaxis, a tetanus toxoid booster and, for some patients, tetanus immune globulin (human) are required.
20. In order to decrease the emergence of vancomycin-resistant enterococci in hospitals and to reduce costs, most clinicians now recommend use of metronidazole first in treatment of patients with *C. difficile* colitis, with oral vancomycin used only for seriously ill patients or those who do not respond to metronidazole.

Infecting Organism	Drug of First Choice	Alternative Drugs
Corynebacterium diphtheriae[21]	erythromycin	penicillin G
Corynebacterium, JK group	vancomycin	penicillin G + gentamicin; erythromycin
**Erysipelothrix rhusiopathiae*	penicillin G	erythromycin, a cephalosporin[5,6], a fluoroquinolone[3]
Listeria monocytogenes	ampicillin ± gentamicin	trimethoprim-sulfamethoxazole
ENTERIC GRAM-NEGATIVE BACILLI		
**Bacteroides*	metronidazole or clindamycin	imipenem; meropenem; ertapenem; amoxicillin/clavulanic acid; ticarcillin/clavulanic acid; piperacillin/tazobactam; ampicillin/sulbactam; cefoxitin[5]; cefotetan[5]; chloramphenicol[16]; penicillin G; gatifloxacin[13] or moxifloxacin[13]
**Campylobacter fetus*	imipenem or meropenem	gentamicin
**Campylobacter jejuni*	erythromycin or azithromycin	a fluoroquinolone[2]; a tetracycline[8]; gentamicin
**Citrobacter freundi*	imipenem or meropenem[22]	a fluoroquinolone[3]; ertapenem; amikacin; a tetracycline[8]; trimethoprim-sulfamethoxazole; cefotaxime[5,22], ceftizoxime[5,22], ceftriaxone[5,22], cefepime[5,22] or ceftazidime[5,22]
**Enterobacter*	imipenem or meropenem[22]	gentamicin, tobramycin or amikacin; trimethoprim-sulfamethoxazole; ciprofloxacin[13]; ticarcillin[23], piperacillin[23]; aztreonam[22]; cefotaxime[5,22], ceftizoxime[5,22], ceftriaxone[5,22], cefepime[5,22] or ceftazidime[5,22]

21. Antitoxin is primary; antimicrobials are used only to halt further toxin production and to prevent the carrier state.
22. In severely ill patients, most Medical Letter consultants would add gentamicin, tobramycin or amikacin.
23. In severely ill patients, most Medical Letter consultants would add gentamicin, tobramycin or amikacin (but see footnote 35).

Infecting Organism	Drug of First Choice	Alternative Drugs
**Escherichia coli*[24]	cefotaxime, ceftizoxime, ceftriaxone, cefepime or ceftazidime[5,22]	ampicillin ± gentamicin, tobramycin or amikacin; ticarcillin[23] or piperacillin[23]; gentamicin, tobramycin or amikacin; amoxicillin/clavulanic acid[22]; ticarcillin/clavulanic acid[23]; piperacillin/tazobactam[23]; ampicillin/sulbactam[22]; trimethoprim-sulfamethoxazole; imipenem[22], meropenem[22], ertapenem[22]; aztreonam[22]; a fluoroquinolone[3]; another cephalosporin[5,6]
**Helicobacter pylori*[25]	omeprazole + amoxicillin + clarithromycin; or tetracycline HCl[8] + metronidazole + bismuth subsalicylate	tetracycline HCl[8] + clarithromycin[11] + bismuth subsalicylate; amoxicillin + metronidazole + bismuth subsalicylate; amoxicillin + clarithromycin[11]
**Klebsiella pneumoniae*[24]	cefotaxime, ceftizoxime, ceftriaxone, cefepime or ceftazidime[5,22]	imipenem[22], meropenem[22], ertapenem[22]; gentamicin, tobramycin or amikacin; amoxicillin/clavulanic acid[22]; ticarcillin/clavulanic acid[23]; piperacillin/tazobactam[23]; ampicillin/sulbactam[22]; trimethoprim-sulfamethoxazole; aztreonam[22]; a fluoroquinolone[3]; piperacillin[23]; another cephalosporin[5,6]

24. For an acute, uncomplicated urinary tract infection, before the infecting organism is known, the drug of first choice is trimethoprim-sulfamethoxazole.
25. Eradication of *H. pylori* with various antibacterial combinations, given concurrently with an H_2-receptor blocker or proton pump inhibitor, has led to rapid healing of active peptic ulcers and low recurrence rates (F Mégraud and B Marshall, Gastroenterol Clin North Am 2000; 29:759).

Infecting Organism	Drug of First Choice	Alternative Drugs
Enteric Gram-Negative Bacilli *(continued)*		
**Proteus mirabilis*[24]	ampicillin[26]	a cephalosporin[5,6,22]; ticarcillin[23], mezlocillin[23] or piperacillin[23]; gentamicin, tobramycin or amikacin; trimethoprim-sulfamethoxazole; imipenem[22], meropenem[22], ertapenem[22]; aztreonam[23]; a fluoroquinolone[3]; chloramphenicol[16]
**Proteus*, indole-positive (including *Providencia rettgeri, Morganella morganii,* and *Proteus vulgaris*)	cefotaxime, ceftizoxime, ceftriaxone, cefepime or ceftazidime[5,22]	imipenem[22], meropenem[22], ertapenem[22]; gentamicin, tobramycin or amikacin; carbenicillin[23], ticarcillin[23], mezlocillin[23] or piperacillin[23]; amoxicillin/clavulanic acid[22]; ticarcillin/clavulanic acid[23]; piperacillin/tazobactam[23]; ampicillin/sulbactam[22]; aztreonam[22]; trimethoprim-sulfamethoxazole; a fluoroquinolone[3]
**Providencia stuartii*	cefotaxime, ceftizoxime, ceftriaxone, cefepime or ceftazidime[5,22]	imipenem[22], meropenem[22], ertapenem[22]; ticarcillin/clavulanic acid[23]; piperacillin/tazobactam[23]; gentamicin, tobramycin or amikacin; carbenicillin[23]; ticarcillin[23], mezlocillin[23] or piperacillin[23]; aztreonam[22]; trimethoprim-sulfamethoxazole; a fluoroquinolone[3]
**Salmonella typhi*[27] (typhoid fever)	a fluoroquinolone[3] or ceftriaxone[5]	chloramphenicol[16]; trimethoprim-sulfamethoxazole; ampicillin; amoxicillin; azithromycin[28]
*other *Salmonella*[29]	cefotaxime[5] or ceftriaxone[5] or a fluoroquinolone[3]	ampicillin or amoxicillin; trimethoprim-sulfamethoxazole; chloramphenicol[16]

26. Large doses (6 grams or more daily) are usually necessary for systemic infections. In severely ill patients, some Medical Letter consultants would add gentamicin, tobramycin or amikacin.
27. A fluoroquinolone or amoxicillin is the drug of choice for *S. typhi* carriers.
28. RW Frenck, Jr et al, Clin Infect Dis 2000; 31:1134.
29. Most cases of *Salmonella* gastroenteritis subside spontaneously without antimicrobial therapy. Immunosuppressed patients, young children and the elderly may benefit the most from antibacterials.

Infecting Organism	Drug of First Choice	Alternative Drugs
**Serratia*	imipenem or meropenem[22]	gentamicin or amikacin; cefotaxime, ceftizoxime, ceftriaxone, cefepime or ceftazidime[5,22]; aztreonam[22]; trimethoprim-sulfamethoxazole; carbenicillin[30], ticarcillin[30] or piperacillin[30]; a fluoroquinolone[3]
**Shigella*	a fluoroquinolone[3]	azithromycin; trimethoprim-sulfamethoxazole; ampicillin; ceftriaxone[5]
**Yersinia enterocolitica*	trimethoprim-sulfamethoxazole	a fluoroquinolone[3]; gentamicin, tobramycin or amikacin; cefotaxime or ceftizoxime[5]
OTHER GRAM-NEGATIVE BACILLI		
**Acinetobacter*	imipenem or meropenem[22]	an aminoglycoside; ciprofloxacin[13]; trimethoprim-sulfamethoxazole; ticarcillin[23] or piperacillin[23]; ceftazidime[22]; minocycline[8]; doxycycline[8]; sulbactam[31]; polymyxin
**Aeromonas*	trimethoprim-sulfamethoxazole	gentamicin or tobramycin; imipenem; a fluoroquinolone[3]
Bartonella henselae or *quintana* (bacillary angiomatosis)	erythromycin	doxycycline[8]; azithromycin
Bartonella henselae[32] (cat scratch bacillus)	azithromycin	ciprofloxacin[13]; erythromycin; trimethoprim-sulfamethoxazole; gentamicin; rifampin
Bordetella pertussis (whooping cough)	erythromycin	azithromycin or clarithromycin[11]; trimethoprim-sulfamethoxazole

30. In severely ill patients, most Medical Letter consultants would add gentamicin or amikacin (but see footnote 35).
31. Sulbactam may be useful to treat multi-drug resistant *Acinetobacter*. It is only available in combination with ampicillin as *Unasyn*. Medical Letter consultants recommend 3 g IV q4h.
32. Role of antibiotics is not clear (DA Conrad, Curr Opin Pediatr 2001; 13:56).

Infecting Organism	Drug of First Choice	Alternative Drugs
Other Gram-Negative Bacilli *(continued)*		
**Brucella*	a tetracycline[8] + rifampin	a tetracycline[8] + streptomycin or gentamicin; chloramphenicol[16] ± streptomycin; trimethoprim-sulfamethoxazole ± gentamicin; ciprofloxacin[13] + rifampin
**Burkholderia cepacia*	trimethoprim-sulfamethoxazole	ceftazidime[5]; chloramphenicol[16]; imipenem
Burkholderia (Pseudomonas) mallei (glanders)	streptomycin + a tetracycline[8]	streptomycin + chloramphenicol[16]; imipenem
**Burkholderia (Pseudomonas) pseudomallei* (melioidosis)	imipenem; ceftazidime[5]	meropenem; chloramphenicol[16] + doxycycline[8] + trimethoprim-sulfamethoxazole; amoxicillin/clavulanic acid
Calymmatobacterium granulomatis (granuloma inguinale)	trimethoprim-sulfamethoxazole	doxycycline[8] or ciprofloxacin[13] ± gentamicin
Capnocytophaga canimorsus[33]	penicillin G	cefotaxime[5]; ceftizoxime[5]; ceftriaxone[5]; imipenem or meropenem; vancomycin; a fluoroquinolone[3]; clindamycin
**Eikenella corrodens*	ampicillin	an erythromycin; a tetracycline[8]; amoxicillin/clavulanic acid; ampicillin/sulbactam; ceftriaxone[5]
**Francisella tularensis* (tularemia)	streptomycin	gentamicin; a tetracycline[8]; chloramphenicol[16]; ciprofloxacin[13]
**Fusobacterium*	penicillin G	metronidazole; clindamycin; cefoxitin[5]; chloramphenicol[16]
Gardnerella vaginalis (bacterial vaginosis)	oral metronidazole[34]	topical clindamycin or metronidazole; oral clindamycin
**Haemophilus ducreyi* (chancroid)	azithromycin or ceftriaxone	ciprofloxacin[13] or erythromycin

33. C Pers et al, Clin Infect Dis 1996; 23:71.
34. Metronidazole is effective for bacterial vaginosis even though it is not usually active *in vitro* against *Gardnerella*.

Infecting Organism	Drug of First Choice	Alternative Drugs
**Haemophilus influenzae*		
meningitis, epiglottitis, arthritis and other serious infections	cefotaxime or ceftriaxone[5]	cefuroxime[5] (not for meningitis); chloramphenicol[16]; meropenem
upper respiratory infections and bronchitis	trimethoprim-sulfamethoxazole	cefuroxime[5]; amoxicillin/clavulanic acid; cefuroxime axetil[5]; cefpodoxime[5]; cefaclor[5]; cefotaxime[5]; ceftizoxime[5]; ceftriaxone[5]; cefixime[5]; a tetracycline[8]; clarithromycin[11]; azithromycin; a fluoroquinolone[3]; ampicillin or amoxicillin
Legionella species	azithromycin or a fluoroquinolone[3] ± rifampin	doxycycline[8] ± rifampin; trimethoprim-sulfamethoxazole; erythromycin
Leptotrichia buccalis	penicillin G	a tetracycline[8]; clindamycin; erythromycin
Pasteurella multocida	penicillin G	a tetracycline[8]; a cephalosporin[5,6]; amoxicillin/clavulanic acid; ampicillin/sulbactam
**Pseudomonas aeruginosa*		
urinary tract infection	ciprofloxacin[13]	levofloxacin[13]; carbenicillin, ticarcillin, piperacillin or mezlocillin; ceftazidime[5]; cefepime[5]; imipenem or meropenem; aztreonam; tobramycin; gentamicin; amikacin
other infections	ticarcillin, mezlocillin or piperacillin + tobramycin, gentamicin or amikacin[35]	ceftazidime,[5] imipenem, meropenem, aztreonam, cefepime[5] + tobramycin, gentamicin or amikacin; ciprofloxacin[13]
Spirillum minus (rat bite fever)	penicillin G	a tetracycline[8]; streptomycin
**Stenotrophomonas maltophilia*	trimethoprim-sulfamethoxazole	minocycline[8]; a fluoroquinolone[3]
Streptobacillus moniliformis (rat bite fever; Haverhill fever)	penicillin G	a tetracycline[8]; streptomycin

* **Resistance may be a problem; susceptibility tests should be used to guide therapy.**

35. Neither gentamicin, tobramycin, netilmicin or amikacin should be mixed in the same bottle with carbenicillin, ticarcillin, mezlocillin or piperacillin for IV administration. When used in high doses or in patients with renal impairment, these penicillins may inactivate the aminoglycosides.

Infecting Organism	Drug of First Choice	Alternative Drugs
Other Gram-Negative Bacilli *(continued)*		
Vibrio cholerae (cholera)[36]	a tetracycline[8]	a fluoroquinolone[3]; trimethoprim-sulfamethoxazole
Vibrio vulnificus	a tetracycline[8]	cefotaxime[5]
Yersinia pestis (plague)	streptomycin ± a tetracycline[8]	chloramphenicol[16]; gentamicin; trimethoprim-sulfamethoxazole
ACID FAST BACILLI		
**Mycobacterium tuberculosis*	isoniazid + rifampin + pyrazinamide ± ethambutol or streptomycin[16]	a fluoroquinolone[3]; cycloserine[16]; capreomycin[16] or kanamycin[16] or amikacin[16]; ethionamide[16]; para-aminosalicylic acid[16]; clofazimine[16]
**Mycobacterium kansasii*	isoniazid + rifampin ± ethambutol or streptomycin[16]	clarithromycin[11] or azithromycin; ethionamide[16]; cycloserine[16]
**Mycobacterium avium* complex	clarithromycin[11] or azithromycin + ethambutol ± rifabutin	ciprofloxacin[13]; amikacin[16]
prophylaxis	clarithromycin[11] or azithromycin ± rifabutin	
**Mycobacterium fortuitum/chelonae* complex	amikacin + clarithromycin[11]	cefoxitin[5]; rifampin; a sulfonamide; doxycycline[8]; ethambutol; linezolid
Mycobacterium marinum (balnei)[37]	minocycline[8]	trimethoprim-sulfamethoxazole; rifampin; clarithromycin[11]; doxycycline[8]
Mycobacterium leprae (leprosy)	dapsone + rifampin ± clofazimine	minocycline[8]; ofloxacin[13]; clarithromycin[11]
ACTINOMYCETES		
Actinomyces israelii (actinomycosis)	penicillin G	a tetracycline[8]; erythromycin; clindamycin
Nocardia	trimethoprim-sulfamethoxazole	sulfisoxazole; amikacin[16]; a tetracycline[8]; imipenem or meropenem; cycloserine[16]; linezolid

36. Antibiotic therapy is an adjunct to and not a substitute for prompt fluid and electrolyte replacement.
37. Most infections are self-limited without drug treatment.

Infecting Organism	Drug of First Choice	Alternative Drugs
**Rhodococcus equi*	vancomycin ± a fluoroquinolone[3], rifampin, imipenem or meropenem; amikacin	erythromycin
Tropheryma whippelii (agent of Whipple's disease)	trimethoprim-sulfamethoxazole	penicillin G; a tetracycline[8]
CHLAMYDIAE		
Chlamydia psittaci (psittacosis; ornithosis)	a tetracycline[8]	chloramphenicol[16]
Chlamydia trachomatis		
(trachoma)	azithromycin	a tetracycline[8] (topical plus oral); a sulfonamide (topical plus oral)
(inclusion conjunctivitis)	erythromycin (oral or IV)	a sulfonamide
(pneumonia)	erythromycin	a sulfonamide
(urethritis, cervicitis)	azithromycin or doxycycline[8]	erythromycin; ofloxacin[13]; amoxicillin
(lymphogranuloma venereum)	a tetracycline[8]	erythromycin
Chlamydia pneumoniae (TWAR strain)	erythromycin; a tetracycline[8]; clarithromycin[11] or azithromycin	a fluoroquinolone[3]
EHRLICHIA		
Ehrlichia chaffeensis	doxycycline[8]	chloramphenicol[16]
Ehrlichia ewingii	doxycycline[8]	
Ehrlichia phagocytophila	doxycycline[8]	rifampin
MYCOPLASMA		
Mycoplasma pneumoniae	erythromycin; a tetracycline[8]; clarithromycin[11] or azithromycin	a fluoroquinolone[3]
Ureaplasma urealyticum	erythromycin	a tetracycline[8]; clarithromycin[11]; azithromycin; ofloxacin[13]

*** Resistance may be a problem; susceptibility tests should be used to guide therapy.**

Infecting Organism	Drug of First Choice	Alternative Drugs
RICKETTSIA — Rocky Mountain spotted fever, endemic typhus (murine), epidemic typhus (louse-borne), scrub typhus, *(Orientia tsutsugamushi)*, trench fever, Q fever	doxycycline[8]	chloramphenicol[16]; a fluoroquinolone[3]; rifampin
SPIROCHETES		
Borrelia burgdorferi (Lyme disease)[38]	doxycycline[8]; amoxicillin; cefuroxime axetil[5]	ceftriaxone[5]; cefotaxime[5]; penicillin G; azithromycin; clarithromycin[11]
Borrelia recurrentis (relapsing fever)	a tetracycline[8]	penicillin G
Leptospira	penicillin G	a tetracycline[8]
Treponema pallidum (syphilis)	penicillin G[10]	a tetracycline[8]; ceftriaxone[5]
Treponema pertenue (yaws)	penicillin G	a tetracycline[8]

38. For treatment of erythema migrans, facial nerve palsy, mild cardiac disease and some cases of arthritis, oral therapy is satisfactory; for more serious neurologic or cardiac disease or arthritis, parenteral therapy with ceftriaxone, cefotaxime or penicillin G is recommended (Medical Letter 2000; 42:37).

COST OF SOME ORAL ANTIBACTERIAL DRUGS

Drug	Dosage[1]	Cost[2]
Azithromycin – *Zithromax*	500 mg day 1, then 250 mg days 2-5	$ 41.94
Cephalosporins		
Cefaclor – average generic	250 mg q8h	35.40
Ceclor		70.05
Ceclor CD	375 mg q12h	84.40
Cefadroxil – average generic	1 gram daily	67.80
Duricef		82.20
Cefdinir – *Omnicef*	300 mg q12h	79.80
Cefditoren – *Spectracef*	200 mg q12h	33.80
Cefixime – *Suprax*	400 mg daily	79.60
Cefpodoxime – *Vantin*	100 mg q12h	67.00
Cefprozil – *Cefzil*	250 mg q12h	70.40
Ceftibuten – *Cedax*	400 mg daily	76.90
Cefuroxime axetil – *Ceftin*	250 mg bid	82.20
Cephalexin – average generic	250 mg q6h	16.00
Keflex		69.20
Keftab	500 mg q12h	67.60
Cephradine – average generic	250 mg q6h	25.20
Velosef		40.40
Loracarbef – *Lorabid*	200 mg q12h	81.00
Clarithromycin – *Biaxin*	250 mg q12h	75.80
Clindamycin – average generic	150 mg q6h	38.80
Cleocin		83.60
Erythromycin		
base, delayed-release capsules	250 mg q6h	
– average generic		11.20
ERYC		23.60
base, enteric-coated tablets	250 mg q6h	
E-Mycin		13.60
Ery-tab		10.40
Fluoroquinolones		
Ciprofloxacin – *Cipro*	250 mg q12h	78.20
Gatifloxacin – *Tequin*	400 mg daily	76.60
Levofloxacin – *Levaquin*	250 mg daily	74.30
Moxifloxacin – *Avelox*	400 mg daily	86.20
Norfloxacin – *Noroxin*	400 mg bid	76.20
Ofloxacin – *Floxin*	200 mg q12h	84.00

(continued)

1. Lowest daily dosage usually recommended.
2. Average cost to the patient for 10 days' treatment (5 days with azithromycin), based on data from retail pharmacies nationwide provided by Scott-Levin's *Source™ Prescription Audit* (SPA), January to December 2001.
3. Each tablet contains 400 mg sulfamethoxazole and 80 mg trimethoprim. Each DS tablet contains 800 mg sulfamethoxazole and 160 mg trimethoprim.

Drug	Dosage[1]	Cost[2]
Fosfomycin – *Monurol*	3 grams once	$ 32.09
Linezolid – *Zyvox*	600 mg q12h	1,055.60
Nitrofurantoin (macrocrystals)	50 mg q6h	
– average generic		8.80
Macrodantin		40.80
Nitrofurantoin monohydrate-macrocrystals	100 mg q12h	
Macrobid		36.60
Penicillins		
Penicillin V – average generic	250 mg q6h	6.40
Veetids		7.20
Amoxicillin – average generic	250 mg q8h	8.40
Amoxil		7.50
Amoxicillin/clavulanic acid		
Augmentin	250 mg q8h	79.20
Ampicillin – average generic	500 mg q6h	11.60
Principen		10.40
Cloxacillin – average generic	500 mg q6h	32.80
Dicloxacillin – average generic	250 mg q6h	15.20
Dycill		18.80
Oxacillin – average generic	500 mg q6h	24.00
Tetracyclines		
Tetracycline HCl – average generic	250 mg q6h	4.40
Sumycin		4.40
Doxycycline	100 mg daily	
capsules – average generic		5.40
Vibramycin		41.40
Trimethoprim-sulfamethoxazole	1 tablet q6h[3]	
– average generic		16.40
Bactrim		38.40
Septra		42.40
double strength (DS) – average generic	1 DS tablet	11.60
Bactrim DS	q12h[3]	31.80
Septra DS		30.00

1. Lowest daily dosage usually recommended.
2. Average cost to the patient for 10 days' treatment (5 days with azithromycin), based on data from retail pharmacies nationwide provided by Scott-Levin's *Source™ Prescription Audit* (SPA), January to December 2001.
3. Each tablet contains 400 mg sulfamethoxazole and 80 mg trimethoprim. Each DS tablet contains 800 mg sulfamethoxazole and 160 mg trimethoprim.

ANTIMICROBIAL PROPHYLAXIS IN SURGERY

Antimicrobial prophylaxis can decrease the incidence of infection, particularly wound infection, after certain operations, but this benefit must be weighed against the risks of toxic and allergic reactions, emergence of resistant bacteria, drug interactions, superinfection and cost (RL Nichols, Emerg Infect Dis 2001; 7:220). Medical Letter consultants generally recommend antimicrobial prophylaxis only for procedures with high infection rates, those involving implantation of prosthetic material and those in which the consequences of infection are especially serious. Recommendations for prevention of surgical site infection and sepsis in surgical patients are listed in the table that begins on page 61. Recommendations for antimicrobial prophylaxis to prevent bacterial endocarditis when patients with prosthetic heart valves, rheumatic heart disease or other cardiac abnormalities undergo dental or surgical procedures are listed on page 64.

CHOICE OF A PROPHYLACTIC AGENT — An effective prophylactic regimen should be directed against the most likely infecting organisms, but need not eradicate every potential pathogen. For most procedures, cefazolin (*Ancef*, and others), which has a moderately long plasma half-life and is active against staphylococci and streptococci, has been effective. For colorectal surgery and appendectomy, cefoxitin *(Mefoxin)* or cefotetan *(Cefotan)* is preferred because they are more active than cefazolin against bowel anaerobes, including *Bacteroides fragilis*. In institutions where methicillin-resistant *Staphylococcus aureus* or methicillin-resistant, coagulase-negative staphylococci are important postoperative pathogens, vancomycin (*Vancocin*, and others) can be used, but routine use of vancomycin for prophylaxis should be discouraged because it may promote emergence of vancomycin-resistant organisms. Long preoperative hospitalizations are associated with increased risk of infection with an antibiotic-resistant organism; local resistance patterns should be taken into account.

Third-generation cephalosporins, such as cefotaxime *(Claforan)*, ceftriaxone *(Rocephin)*, cefoperazone *(Cefobid)*, ceftazidime *(Fortaz*, and others), or ceftizoxime *(Cefizox)*, and fourth-generation cephalosporins such as cefepime *(Maxipime)* should not be used for routine surgical prophylaxis because they are expensive, some are less active than cefazolin against staphylococci, their spectrum of activity includes organisms rarely encountered in elective surgery, and their widespread use for prophylaxis may promote emergence of resistance.

NUMBER OF DOSES — In most instances, a single intravenous dose of an antimicrobial completed 30 minutes or less before the skin incision provides adequate tissue concentrations throughout the operation. If surgery is prolonged (more than four hours), major blood loss occurs or an antimicrobial with a short half-life (such as cefoxitin) is used, administration of one or more additional doses may be advisable during the procedure. Published studies of antimicrobial prophylaxis often use one or two doses postoperatively in addition to one dose just before surgery. Most Medical Letter consultants believe, however, that postoperative doses are usually unnecessary.

CARDIAC — Prophylactic antibiotics can decrease the incidence of infection after cardiac surgery (I Kriaras et al, Eur J Cardiothorac Surg 2000; 18:440). A meta-analysis of seven placebo-controlled randomized studies of antimicrobial prophylaxis for implantation of permanent pacemakers showed a statistically significant reduction in the incidence of infection (A DaCosta et al, Circulation 1998; 97:1796).

GASTROINTESTINAL — Antibiotic prophylaxis is recommended for esophageal surgery in the presence of obstruction, which increases the risk of infection. The risk of infection after gastroduodenal surgery is high when gastric acidity and gastrointestinal motility are diminished by obstruction, hemorrhage, gastric ulcer or malignancy, or by therapy with an H_2-blocker such as ranitidine (*Zantac*, and others) or a proton pump inhibitor such as omeprazole *(Prilosec)*, and is also high in patients with morbid obesity. A dose of cefazolin or cefoxitin given 30 minutes before surgery can decrease the incidence of postoperative infection in these circumstances. Prophylactic antibiotics are not indicated for routine gastroesophageal endoscopy, but some clinicians use them for high-risk patients undergoing esophageal dilatation or sclerotherapy of varices, and most use them before placement of a percutaneous gastrostomy (D Külling et al, Gastrointest Endosc 2000; 51:152; VK Sharma et al, Am J Gastroenterol 2000; 95:3133).

Antimicrobials are recommended before biliary tract surgery for patients with a high risk of infection — those more than 70 years old and those with acute cholecystitis, a non-functioning gallbladder, obstructive jaundice or common duct stones. Many clinicians follow similar guidelines for antibiotic prophylaxis of endoscopic retrograde cholangiopancreatography (ERCP). Prophylactic antibiotics are not necessary for low-risk patients undergoing elective laparoscopic cholecystectomy (KJ Dobay et al, Ann Surg 1999; 65:226; A Higgins et al, Arch Surg 1999; 134:611).

Preoperative antibiotics can decrease the incidence of infection after colorectal surgery; for elective operations, an oral regimen of neomycin and erythromycin appears to be as effective as parenteral drugs. Many surgeons in North America use a combination of oral and parenteral agents, but it is unclear if this is more effective than either alone. Preoperative antimicrobials can decrease the incidence of infection after surgery for acute appendicitis. If perforation has occurred, antibiotics should be considered therapeutic and continued as long as clinically indicated.

GYNECOLOGY AND OBSTETRICS — Antimicrobial prophylaxis decreases the incidence of infection after vaginal and abdominal hysterectomy (V Tanos and N Rojansky, J Am Coll Surg 1994; 179:593; AA Kamat et al, Infect Dis Obstet Gynecol 2000; 8:230). Peri- or preoperative antimicrobials can prevent infection when given after cord clamping in emergency cesarean section, in high-risk situations such as active labor or premature rupture of membranes, after first-trimester abortion in high-risk women, and after mid-trimester abortions (D Chelmow et al, Am J Obstet Gynecol 2001; 184:656). One meta-analysis found a protective effect of perioperative antibacterials in all women undergoing therapeutic abortion (GF Sawaya et al, Obstet Gynecol 1996; 87:884).

HEAD AND NECK — Prophylaxis with antimicrobials has decreased the incidence of surgical site infection after head and neck operations that involve an incision through the oral or pharyngeal mucosa (RS Weber, Ear Nose Throat J 1997; 76:790; JP Rodrigo et al, Head Neck 1997; 19:188).

NEUROSURGERY — Studies of antimicrobial prophylaxis for implantation of permanent cerebrospinal fluid shunts have produced conflicting results (EM Brown et al, Lancet 1994; 344:1547). An antistaphylococcal antibiotic can decrease the incidence of infection after craniotomy. In spinal surgery, the post-operative infection rate after conventional lumbar discectomy is low, and antibiotics have generally not been shown to be effective; infection rates are higher after spinal procedures involving fusion, prolonged spinal surgery or insertion of foreign material, and prophylactic antibiotics are often used, but controlled trials demonstrating their effectiveness are lacking (JB Dimick et al, Spine 2000; 25:2544). Despite the low risk of infection, the serious consequences of surgical site infection have led many neurosurgeons to use perioperative antibiotics.

OPHTHALMIC — Data are limited on the effectiveness of antimicrobial prophylaxis for ophthalmic surgery, but postoperative endophthalmitis can be devastating (TA Ciulla et al, Ophthalmol 2002; 109:13). Most ophthalmologists use antimicrobial eye drops for prophylaxis, and some also give a subconjunctival injection. There is no consensus supporting a particular choice, route or duration of antimicrobial prophylaxis (TJ Liesegang, Cornea 1999; 18:383). There is no evidence that prophylactic antibiotics are needed for procedures that do not invade the globe.

ORTHOPEDIC — Prophylactic antistaphylococcal drugs administered preoperatively can decrease the incidence of both early and late infection following joint replacement. They also decrease the rate of infection in compound or open fractures and when hip and other fractures are treated with internal fixation by nails, plates, screws or wires. One large randomized trial found a single dose of a cephalosporin more effective than placebo in preventing wound infection after surgical repair of closed fractures (H Boxma et al,

Lancet 1996; 347:1133). A prospective randomized study in patients undergoing diagnostic and operative arthroscopic surgery concluded that antibiotic prophylaxis is not indicated (JA Wieck et al, Orthopedics 1997; 20:133).

THORACIC (NON-CARDIAC) — Antibiotic prophylaxis is given routinely in pulmonary surgery, but supporting data are sparse. In one study, a single preoperative dose of cefazolin after pulmonary resection led to a decrease in the incidence of surgical site infection, but not of pneumonia or empyema. Other trials have found that multiple doses of a cephalosporin can prevent infection after closed-tube thoracostomy for chest trauma (RP Gonzalez and MR Holevar, Am Surg 1998; 64:617). Insertion of chest tubes for other indications, such as spontaneous pneumothorax, does not require antimicrobial prophylaxis.

UROLOGY —Infectious disease experts do not recommend antimicrobials before most urological operations in patients with sterile urine. When the urine culture is positive or unavailable, or the patient has a preoperative urinary catheter, patients should be treated to sterilize the urine before surgery or receive a single preoperative dose of an appropriate agent (CM Kunin, *Urinary Tract Infections: Detection, Prevention and Management*, 5th ed, Baltimore:Williams & Wilkins, 1997, p 363). Prophylaxis is recommended before transrectal prostatic biopsies because urosepsis has occurred (HM Taylor and JB Bingham, J Antimicrob Chemother 1997; 39:115).

VASCULAR — Preoperative administration of a cephalosporin decreases the incidence of postoperative surgical site infection after arterial reconstructive surgery on the abdominal aorta, vascular operations on the leg that include a groin incision, and amputation of the lower extremity for ischemia (Swedish-Norwegian Consensus Group, Scand J Infect Dis 1998; 30:547). Many experts also recommend prophylaxis for implantation of any vascular prosthetic material, such as grafts for vascular access in hemodialysis. Prophylaxis is not indicated for carotid endarterectomy or brachial artery repair without prosthetic material.

OTHER PROCEDURES —The small number of surgical site infections that would be prevented by antimicrobial prophylaxis make it unwarranted for cardiac catheterization, varicose vein surgery, most dermatologic and plastic surgery, arterial puncture, thoracentesis, paracentesis, repair of simple lacerations, outpatient treatment of burns, dental extractions or root canal therapy. The need for prophylaxis in breast surgery, herniorraphy and other "clean" surgical procedures has been controversial (SL Gorbach, Infect Dis Clin Pract 1999; 8:1; R Gupta et al, Eur J Surg Oncol 2000; 26:363). Medical Letter consultants generally do not recommend surgical prophylaxis for these procedures because of the low rate of infection in many hospitals, the low morbidity of these infections and the potential adverse effects of using prophylaxis in such a large number of patients.

CONTAMINATED ("DIRTY") SURGERY — "Dirty" surgery, such as that for a perforated abdominal viscus, a compound fracture or a laceration due to an animal or human bite, is often followed by infection. Use of antimicrobial drugs for these operations is considered therapy rather than prophylaxis and should be continued postoperatively for several days.

PATIENTS WITH PROSTHETIC JOINTS — Patients with prosthetic joints generally do not require antimicrobial prophylaxis when undergoing dental, gastrointestinal or genitourinary procedures (J Segreti, Infect Dis Clin North Am 1999; 13:871). For long procedures, surgery in an infected area (including periodontal disease) or other procedures with a high risk of bacteremia, and possibly for selected patients at high risk for infection, prophylaxis may be advisable (American Dental Association and American Academy of Orthopaedic Surgeons, J Am Dent Assoc 1997; 128:1).

PATIENTS WITH PENICILLIN ALLERGY — Cefazolin is often used for prophylaxis in penicillin-allergic patients, but such patients may also have allergic reactions to cephalosporins. When allergy prevents the use of a cephalosporin, vancomycin or clindamycin can be used but neither is effective against gram-negative bacteria; in such patients, some Medical Letter consultants would add another agent such as ciprofloxacin to cover gram-negative bacteria depending on the site of surgery and the procedure.

CHOICE OF DRUG FOR PREVENTION OF SURGICAL SITE INFECTION

Nature of operation	Likely pathogens	Recommended drugs	Adult dosage before surgery[1]
Cardiac			
Prosthetic valve, coronary artery bypass, other open-heart surgery, pacemaker or defibrillator implant	*Staphylococcus aureus, S. epidermidis, Corynebacterium*, enteric gram-negative bacilli	cefazolin or cefuroxime *OR* vancomycin[3]	1-2 grams IV[2] 1.5 grams IV[2] 1 gram IV
Gastrointestinal			
Esophageal, gastroduodenal	Enteric gram-negative bacilli, gram-positive cocci	*High risk*[4] only: cefazolin[5]	 1-2 grams IV
Biliary tract	Enteric gram-negative bacilli, enterococci, clostridia	*High risk*[6] *only:* cefazolin[5]	 1-2 grams IV
Colorectal	Enteric gram-negative bacilli, anaerobes, enterococci	*Oral:* neomycin + erythromycin base[7]	
		Parenteral:	
		cefoxitin	1-2 grams IV
		or cefotetan	1-2 grams IV
		OR cefazolin	1-2 grams IV
		+ metronidazole	0.5 grams IV

1. Parenteral prophylactic antimicrobials can be given as a single IV dose completed 30 minutes or less before the operation. For prolonged operations, additional intraoperative doses should be given q4-8h for the duration of the procedure.
2. Some consultants recommend an additional dose when patients are removed from bypass during open-heart surgery.
3. For hospitals in which methicillin-resistant *S. aureus* and *S. epidermidis* are a frequent cause of postoperative wound infection, or for patients allergic to penicillins or cephalosporins. Rapid IV administration may cause hypotension, which could be especially dangerous during induction of anesthesia. Even if the drug is given over 60 minutes, hypotension may occur; treatment with diphenhydramine (*Benadryl*, and others) and further slowing of the infusion rate may be helpful. For procedures in which enteric gram-negative bacilli are likely pathogens, such as vascular surgery involving a groin incision, cefazolin or cefuroxime should be included in the prophylaxis regimen for patients not allergic to cephalosporins.
4. Morbid obesity, esophageal obstruction, decreased gastric acidity or gastrointestinal motility.
5. Some Medical Letter consultants favor cefoxitin for better anaerobic coverage in this setting.
6. Age >70 years, acute cholecystitis, non-functioning gall bladder, obstructive jaundice or common duct stones.
7. After appropriate diet and catharsis, 1 g of each at 1 PM, 2 PM and 11 PM the day before an 8 AM operation.

Nature of operation	Likely pathogens	Recommended drugs	Adult dosage before surgery[1]
Appendectomy, non-perforated	Enteric gram-negative bacilli, anaerobes, enterococci	cefoxitin or cefotetan	1-2 grams IV 1-2 grams IV
Genitourinary	Enteric gram-negative bacilli, enterococci	*High risk[8] only:* ciprofloxacin	500 mg PO or 400 mg IV
Gynecologic and Obstetric			
Vaginal or abdominal hysterectomy	Enteric gram-negatives, anaerobes, Gp B strep, enterococci	cefazolin or cefotetan or cefoxitin	1-2 grams IV 1-2 grams IV 1 gram IV
Cesarean section	same as for hysterectomy	*High risk[9] only:* cefazolin	1 gram IV after cord clamping
Abortion	same as for hysterectomy	*First trimester, high risk[10]:* aqueous penicillin G *OR* doxycycline *Second trimester:* cefazolin	2 mill units IV 300 mg PO[11] 1 gram IV
Head and Neck Surgery			
Incisions through oral or pharyngeal mucosa	Anaerobes, enteric gram-negative bacilli, *S. aureus*	clindamycin + gentamicin OR cefazolin	600-900 mg IV 1.5 mg/kg IV 1-2 grams IV
Neurosurgery			
Craniotomy	*S. aureus, S. epidermidis*	cefazolin *OR* vancomycin[3]	1-2 grams IV 1 gram IV
Ophthalmic	*S. epidermidis, S. aureus,* streptococci, enteric gram-negative bacilli, *Pseudomonas*	gentamicin, tobramycin, ciprofloxacin, ofloxacin or neomycin-gramicidin-polymyxin B cefazolin	multiple drops topically over 2 to 24 hours 100 mg subconjunctivally

8. Urine culture positive or unavailable, preoperative catheter, transrectal prostatic biopsy.
9. Active labor or premature rupture of membranes.
10. Patients with previous pelvic inflammatory disease, previous gonorrhea or multiple sex partners.
11. Divided into 100 mg one hour before the abortion and 200 mg one half hour after.

Nature of operation	Likely pathogens	Recommended drugs	Adult dosage before surgery[1]
Orthopedic			
Total joint replacement, internal fixation of fractures	*S. aureus, S. epidermidis*	cefazolin *OR* vancomycin[3]	1-2 grams IV 1 gram IV
Thoracic (Non-Cardiac)	*S. aureus, S. epidermidis,* streptococci, enteric gram-negative bacilli	cefazolin or cefuroxime *OR* vancomycin[3]	1-2 grams IV 1.5 grams IV 1 gram IV
Vascular			
Arterial surgery involving a prosthesis, the abdominal aorta, or a groin incision	*S. aureus, S. epidermidis,* enteric gram-negative bacilli	cefazolin *OR* vancomycin[3]	1-2 grams IV 1 gram IV
Lower extremity amputation for ischemia	*S. aureus, S. epidermidis,* enteric gram-negative bacilli, clostridia	cefazolin[5] *OR* vancomycin[3]	1-2 grams IV 1 gram IV
CONTAMINATED SURGERY[12]			
Ruptured viscus	Enteric gram-negative bacilli, anaerobes, enterococci	cefoxitin or cefotetan ± gentamicin *OR* clindamycin + gentamicin	1-2 g IV q6h 1-2 g IV q12h 1.5 mg/kg IV q8h 600 mg IV q6h 1.5 mg/kg IV q8h
Traumatic wound	*S. aureus,* Gp A strep, clostridia	cefazolin[13]	1-2 grams IV q8h

12. For contaminated or "dirty" surgery, therapy should usually be continued for about five days. Ruptured viscus in postoperative setting (dehiscence) requires antibacterials to include coverage of nosocomial pathogens.
13. For bite wounds, in which likely pathogens may also include oral anaerobes, *Eikenella corrodens* (human), or *Pasteurella multocida* (dog and cat), some Medical Letter consultants recommend use of amoxicillin/clavulanic acid *(Augmentin)* or ampicillin/sulbactam *(Unasyn)* (PF Smith et al, J Clin Pharm Ther 2000; 25:85). For penetrating intracranial wounds, including gunshot injuries, a broad-spectrum antimicrobial such as ampicillin/sulbactam is recommended (R Bayston et al, Lancet 2000; 355:1813).

PREVENTION OF BACTERIAL ENDOCARDITIS

Many physicians believe that antimicrobial prophylaxis before procedures that may cause transient bacteremia can prevent endocarditis in patients with valvular heart disease, prosthetic heart valves or other structural cardiac abnormalities. The effectiveness of this common practice has never been established by controlled trials in humans (G Hall et al, Clin Infect Dis 1999; 29:1). The drugs and dosages in the table are based on those recommended by the American Heart Association (AS Dajani et al, JAMA 1997; 277:1794).

ENDOCARDITIS PROPHYLAXIS[1]

	Dosage for Adults	Dosage for Children*
DENTAL AND UPPER RESPIRATORY PROCEDURES[2]		
Oral		
Amoxicillin[3] (*Amoxil*, and others)	2 grams 1 hour before procedure	50 mg/kg 1 hour before procedure
Penicillin allergy:		
Clindamycin (*Cleocin*, and others)	600 mg 1 hour before procedure	20 mg/kg 1 hour before procedure
OR		
Cephalexin** (*Keflex*, and others) or Cefadroxil** (*Duricef*, and others)	2 grams 1 hour before procedure	50 mg/kg 1 hour before procedure
OR		
Azithromycin (*Zithromax*) or Clarithromycin (*Biaxin*)	500 mg 1 hour before procedure	15 mg/kg 1 hour before procedure
Parenteral (for patients unable to take oral drugs)		
Ampicillin (*Omnipen*, and others)	2 grams IM or IV within 30 minutes before procedure	50 mg/kg IM or IV within 30 minutes before procedure
Penicillin allergy:		
Clindamycin	600 mg IV within 30 minutes before procedure	20 mg/kg IV within 30 minutes before procedure
OR		
Cefazolin** (*Ancef*, and others)	1 gram IM or IV within 30 minutes before procedure	25 mg/kg IM or IV within 30 minutes before procedure

	Dosage for Adults	Dosage for Children*
GASTROINTESTINAL AND GENITOURINARY PROCEDURES[2]		
Oral		
Amoxicillin[3]	2 grams 1 hour before procedure	50 mg/kg 1 hour before procedure
Parenteral		
Ampicillin[4]	2 grams IM or IV within 30 minutes before procedure	50 mg/kg IM or IV within 30 minutes before procedure
± Gentamicin[5] (*Garamycin*, and others)	1.5 mg/kg (120 mg max.) IM or IV within 30 minutes before procedure	1.5 mg/kg IM or IV within 30 minutes before procedure
Penicillin allergy:		
Vancomycin (*Vancocin*, and others)	1 gram IV infused *slowly over 1 hour* beginning 1 hour before procedure	20 mg/kg IV infused *slowly over 1 hour* beginning 1 hour before procedure
± Gentamicin[5]	1.5 mg/kg (120 mg max.) IM or IV within 30 minutes before procedure	1.5 mg/kg IM or IV within 30 minutes before procedure

* Should not exceed adult dosage

** Not recommended for patients with history of recent, severe or immediate-type (urticaria, angioedema, anaphylaxis) allergy to penicillin.

1. The risk of endocarditis is considered high in patients with previous endocarditis, prosthetic heart valves, complex cyanotic congenital heart disease such as tetralogy of Fallot, or surgically constructed systemic pulmonary shunts or conduits. The risk is also considered worth treating in patients with other forms of congenital heart disease (but not uncomplicated secundum atrial septal defect), acquired (such as rheumatic) valvular disease, hypertrophic cardiomyopathy, and mitral valve prolapse with regurgitation or thickened leaflets. Viridans streptococci are the most common cause of endocarditis after dental or upper respiratory procedures; enterococci are the most common cause after gastrointestinal or genitourinary procedures.
2. For a review of the risk of bacteremia with various procedures, see AS Dajani et al, JAMA 1997; 277:1794. Among dental procedures, some experts believe that tooth extractions and gingival surgery, including implant placement, have the highest risk of endocarditis (DT Durack, Ann Intern Med 1998; 129:829).
3. Amoxicillin is recommended because of its excellent bioavailability and good activity against streptococci and enterococci.
4. High-risk patients given parenteral ampicillin before the procedure should receive a dose of ampicillin 1 gram IM or IV or a dose of amoxicillin 1 gram orally six hours afterwards.
5. Gentamicin should be added for patients with a high risk of endocarditis (see footnote 1).

DRUGS FOR TUBERCULOSIS

Tuberculosis (TB) is still a problem in the United States, even though the incidence continues to decline. Poor adherence to therapy is the most important cause of treatment failure and is associated with emergence of drug resistance. Medical Letter consultants now recommend that most patients take drugs for TB under direct observation ("directly observed therapy" or DOT). DOT services are available through local and state health department TB programs.

TREATMENT OF ACTIVE TB — All isolates of *Mycobacterium tuberculosis* should be tested for antimicrobial susceptibility, but results generally do not become available for at least 2 weeks and sometimes much longer (CR Horsburgh, Jr, et al, Clin Infect Dis 2000; 31:633). For empiric initial treatment in most areas of the US, experts generally recommend an initial 4-drug combination of isoniazid, rifampin, pyrazinamide and either ethambutol or streptomycin (PM Small and PI Fujiwara, N Engl J Med 2001; 345:189). For patients with disseminated TB, tuberculous osteomyelitis or TB meningitis, Medical Letter consultants recommend continuing treatment for at least 9 months, and for 12 months in children.

Susceptible Organisms – When the patient has TB caused by a fully susceptible strain, isoniazid, rifampin and pyrazinamide can be given for the first 2 months, followed by isoniazid and rifampin (without pyrazinamide) for the next 4 months to complete 6 months of therapy. Among all the drugs used for treatment of TB, effectiveness is best documented for isoniazid and rifampin taken daily, or 2 or 3 times a week. A regimen containing only isoniazid and rifampin given for 9 months is effective for fully susceptible organisms in patients who cannot take pyrazinamide, such as pregnant women.

Alternative regimens for patients who cannot tolerate rifampin include isoniazid plus ethambutol for 18 months (preferably with streptomycin for the first 2 months), 12 months of isoniazid, ethambutol, a fluoroquinolone (such as levofloxacin) and pyrazinamide, or 9 months of isoniazid, ethambutol, pyrazinamide, and streptomycin (for the first 2 months), with or without a fluoroquinolone throughout.

Resistance to Isoniazid – Tuberculosis resistant only to isoniazid (the most common form of resistance) can be treated with rifampin, pyrazinamide and either ethambutol or streptomycin for 6 months (or, for patients who cannot tolerate pyrazinamide, with rifampin and ethambutol for 12 months).

Multidrug-Resistant Organisms – Multidrug-resistant (MDR) TB (resistant at least to isoniazid and rifampin) should be treated with 4 or more drugs to which the organism is susceptible. Due to the complexity and duration of treatment regimens, Medical Letter consultants recommend daily DOT and consultation with clinicians experienced with the treatment of MDRTB. Treatment should be continued for 18 to 24 months, or 12 months after the culture becomes negative. When MDRTB is likely, or in patients with a history of previous treatment for TB, some clinicians now start with combinations of 5, 6 or 7 drugs before laboratory susceptibility data are available. Typically, empiric therapy for suspected MDRTB includes isoniazid, rifampin, ethambutol, pyrazinamide, an aminoglycoside (streptomycin, kanamycin or amikacin) or capreomycin, a fluoroquinolone such as levofloxacin, and either cycloserine, ethionamide or aminosalicylic acid (PAS).

Intermittent Treatment – Intermittent high-dose, 4-drug regimens with 3 doses per week from the outset or 2 doses per week after at least 2 weeks of daily therapy can also be effective for treatment of some cases of TB. Medical Letter consultants strongly recommend DOT for all intermittent regimens. Intermittent treatment should not be used for treatment of MDRTB.

Fixed-Dose Combinations – A combination formulation of rifampin 120 mg, isoniazid 50 mg and pyrazinamide 300 mg *(Rifater)* is approved by the FDA for the initial 2 months of daily anti-tuberculosis therapy. The dosage is 4 tablets once each day for patients weighing ≤44 kg, 5 tablets for 45 to 54 kg and 6 tablets for ≥55 kg. A combination of rifampin 300 mg and isoniazid 150 mg *(Rifamate)* has been available in the US since 1975. Fixed-dose combinations may be particularly useful for patients taking drugs themselves and not under direct observation.

HIV-INFECTED PATIENTS NOT ON HAART — For HIV-infected patients requiring treatment for TB who are not currently being treated with highly active anti-retroviral therapy (HAART), it may be prudent to delay HAART for 2 or more months in order to avoid a paradoxical worsening of TB due to immune reconstitution, as well as decrease the risk of overlapping drug adverse effects and interactions, and to enhance adherence to both drug regimens (WJ Burman and BE Jones, Am J Respir Crit Care Med 2001; 164:7).

HIV-INFECTED PATIENTS ON HAART — Rifampin accelerates the metabolism of protease inhibitors and some non-nucleoside reverse transcriptase inhibitors, decreasing their serum concentrations, possibly to ineffective levels. In addition, protease inhibitors slow metabolism of rifabutin, increasing serum concentrations and possibly toxicity.

Standard 4-drug treatment including rifampin can be used in HIV-infected patients with active TB who are simultaneously receiving HAART if the HAART regimen consists of efavirenz *(Sustiva)* and two nucleoside reverse transcriptase inhibitors (NRTIs). Rifampin can also be used in patients taking ritonavir *(Norvir)* plus two NRTIs or a combination of ritonavir and saquinavir (MMWR Morb Mortal Wkly Rep 2000; 49:185).

For patients on other HAART regimens, there are two alternatives. The first is to substitute low-dose rifabutin (150 mg qd) for rifampin in the standard regimen (i.e., isoniazid, rifabutin, pyrazinamide and ethambutol) and use indinavir *(Crixivan)*, nelfinavir *(Viracept)* or amprenavir *(Agenerase)* as the protease inhibitor. Rifabutin appears to be as effective as rifampin against TB, and has less effect on protease inhibitor levels, at least with these three protease inhibitors. If the HAART regimen contains nevirapine *(Viramune)*, the usual dose of rifabutin (300 mg daily) should be used. Higher rifabutin doses (450-600 mg daily) are needed if the HAART regimen contains efavirenz. A less effective alternative for HIV-infected patients on HAART is to use a non-rifamycin containing regimen such as isoniazid, pyrazinamide and ethambutol for 9 months with streptomycin for the first 2 months (MMWR Morb Mortal Wkly Rep 1998; 47, RR-20:1).

ADVERSE EFFECTS — Serum aminotransferase activity increases in 10% to 20% of patients taking **isoniazid**, especially in the early weeks of treatment, but often returns to normal even when the drug is continued. Severe liver damage due to isoniazid is more likely to occur in patients more than 35 years old, but can also occur in younger patients. Medical Letter consultants recommend stopping isoniazid when serum aspartate aminotransferase activity reaches five times the upper limit of normal or if the patient has symptoms of hepatitis, but it can sometimes be re-started later. Peripheral neuropathy occurs rarely but can be prevented by supplementation with pyridoxine (10-25 mg/day), which is recommended for patients with chronic alcohol use, diabetes, chronic renal failure, HIV infection, and for pregnant women and malnourished patients.

Rifampin is also potentially hepatotoxic, and gastrointestinal disturbances, rash and thrombocytopenic purpura can occur. Whenever possible, rifampin should be continued despite minor adverse reactions such as pruritus and gastrointestinal upset. When taken erratically, the drug can cause a febrile "flu-like" syndrome and, very rarely, shortness of breath, hemolytic anemia, shock and acute renal failure. Patients should be warned that rifampin may turn urine, tears and other body fluids reddish-orange and can permanently stain contact lenses and lens implants. Rifampin can also increase the metabolism and decrease the effect of many other drugs, including systemic contraceptives, corticosteroids, warfarin, quinidine, methadone (*Dolophine*, and others), delavirdine *(Rescriptor)*, clarithromycin (*Biaxin*), ketoconazole *(Nizoral)*, itraconazole *(Sporanox)* and fluconazole *(Diflucan)*, as well as protease inhibitors (*Medical Letter Handbook of Adverse Drug Interactions*, 2002, page 430). **Rifabutin** and **rifapentine**, a long-acting analog of rifampin, have similar adverse effects;

rifabutin can also cause uveitis, skin hyperpigmentation and a lupus-like syndrome, but is less likely than rifampin to interact with other drugs.

Pyrazinamide often causes morbilliform rash, arthralgias and hyperuricemia (clinical gout is rare), and blocks the hypouricemic action of allopurinol (*Zyloprim*, and others). Gastrointestinal disturbances and hepatotoxicity can occur. **Ethambutol** can cause optic neuritis, but rarely with a dosage of 15 mg/kg daily. It is usually not recommended for children too young to have visual acuity monitored. **Streptomycin** causes ototoxicity, usually vestibular disturbances, and, less frequently, renal toxicity. **Amikacin, kanamycin** and **capreomycin** can cause nephro-, oto- and vestibular toxicity. **Cycloserine** can cause psychiatric symptoms and seizures. **Ethionamide** has been associated with gastrointestinal, hepatic and thyroid toxicity. A delayed-release formulation of **aminosalicylic acid** (PAS, *Paser)* may be better tolerated than older formulations. **Fluoroquinolones** are usually well-tolerated but can cause gastrointestinal and CNS disturbances.

TREATMENT OF LATENT TB INFECTION — The risk of developing clinical tuberculosis is greatest in patients also infected with HIV or receiving immunosuppressive therapy, in close contacts of those with recent pulmonary tuberculosis, in patients with X-ray evidence of prior TB, in the first 2 years after development of a positive tuberculin test, and in recent immigrants. The risk of serious disease, including miliary tuberculosis and tuberculous meningitis, is highest in infants, the elderly and in patients with HIV infection or other causes of severe immunosuppression. Tuberculin skin testing and treatment of latent TB infection is most important in these patients.

Isoniazid is generally the drug of choice for treatment of latent TB infection (ATS/CDC, Am J Respir Crit Care Med 2000; 161:S221). It should be given for 9 months in a single daily dose of 300 mg for adults and 10 mg/kg (maximum 300 mg/day) for children or with DOT as 900 mg twice a week for adults or 20 mg/kg for children (MMWR Morb Mortal Wkly Rep 2000; 49 RR-6:1). It is probably safe for treatment of latent TB in pregnancy (G Bothamley, Drug Saf 2001; 24:553).

Other possible regimens for treatment of latent TB include daily rifampin alone for 4 months or rifampin and pyrazinamide for 2 months. These regimens may be useful in persons found to be tuberculin-positive after exposure to patients with organisms resistant to isoniazid. However, recent data suggest a risk of potentially lethal hepatotoxicity with the rifampin and pyrazinamide regimen and most Medical Letter consultants would limit its use (MMWR Morb Mortal Wkly Rep 2001, 50:738; WJ Burman and RR Reves, Am J Respir Crit Care Med 2001; 164:1112). For patients with a known exposure to MDRTB and a high risk of developing active TB (eg, HIV-infected), regimens with two drugs to which the organism is susceptible such as pyrazinamide plus ethambutol for 9 to 12 months or pyrazinamide plus a fluoroquinolone for 6 to 12 months can be used, but these may be poorly tolerated (R Ridzon et al, Clin Infect Dis 1997; 24:1264).

CONCLUSION — All isolates of *M. tuberculosis* should be tested for antimicrobial susceptibility. Initial therapy for most patients with active TB should include at least isoniazid, a rifamycin, pyrazinamide, and either ethambutol or streptomycin until susceptibility is known. When therapy is not directly observed by a health care worker, use of the fixed-dose combinations *Rifamate* and *Rifater* may improve compliance and prevent emergence of drug resistance. Confirmed multidrug-resistant tuberculosis should be treated under DOT with at least 4 drugs to which the organism is susceptible; the total duration of therapy usually is 18 to 24 months, or 12 months after the culture becomes negative.

(Continues on next page)

SOME ANTITUBERCULOSIS DRUGS

Drug	Adult dosage (daily)	Pediatric dosage (daily)	Main adverse effects
Isoniazid (INH)[1,2]	300 mg PO, IM	10-20 mg/kg (max. 300 mg)	Hepatic toxicity, peripheral neuropathy
Rifampin[1,3] *(Rifadin, Rimactane)*	600 mg PO, IV	10-20 mg/kg (max. 600 mg)	Hepatic toxicity, flu-like syndrome
Rifabutin[4] *(Mycobutin)*	300 mg/day	5 mg/kg[5]	Hepatic toxicity, flu-like syndrome, iritis
Rifapentine *(Priftin)*[5]	600 mg PO[6]	No data available	Hepatic toxicity, hyperuricemia
Pyrazinamide[7]	1.5 to 2.5 g PO	15-30 mg/kg (max. 2 g)	Arthralgias, hepatic toxicity, hyperuricemia
Ethambutol[8] *(Myambutol)*	15-25 mg/kg PO	15-25 mg/kg	Optic neuritis
Streptomycin[9]	15 mg/kg IM	20-30 mg/kg	Vestibular and auditory toxicity, renal damage

1. An intravenous preparation is available.
2. For intermittent use after a few weeks to months of daily therapy, dosage is 15 mg/kg (max. 900 mg) twice/week for adults. Pyridoxine 10 to 25 mg should be given to prevent neuropathy in malnourished or pregnant patients and those with HIV infection, alcoholism or diabetes.
3. For intermittent use after a few weeks to months of daily therapy, dosage is 600 mg twice/week.
4. For intermittent use after a few weeks to months of daily therapy, dosage is 300 mg 2 or 3 times a week. For use with amprenavir, nelfinavir or indinavir, the rifabutin dose is 150 mg/day or 300 mg 2-3 times a week. For use with efavirenz, the rifabutin dose is increased to 450-600 mg/day or 600 mg 2-3 times a week. No dose adjustment is needed in use with nevirapine.
5. No pediatric formulation available.
6. For intermittent use, 600 mg twice a week for first two months, followed by 600 mg once a week. Rifamycin resistance has been reported in HIV-infected patients treated with weekly isoniazid and rifapentine (A Vernon et al, Lancet 1999; 353:1843).
7. For intermittent use after a few weeks to months of daily therapy, dosage is 2.5 to 3.5 g twice/week.
8. Usually not recommended for children when visual acuity cannot be monitored. Some clinicians use 25 mg/kg/day during first one or two months or longer if organism is isoniazid-resistant. Decrease dosage if renal function diminished. For intermittent use after a few weeks to months of daily therapy, dosage is 50 mg/kg twice/week.
9. When oral drugs are given daily, streptomycin is generally given 5 times per week (15 mg/kg, or a maximum of 1 g per dose) for an initial 2 to 12 week period, and then (if needed) 2 to 3 times per week (20 to 30 mg/kg, or a maximum of 1.5 g per dose). For patients > 40 years old, dosage is reduced to 500 to 750 mg 5 times per week and 20 mg/kg when given twice per week. Some clinicians change to lower dosage at 60 rather than 40 years old. Dosage should be decreased if renal function is diminished.

Drug	Adult dosage (daily)	Pediatric dosage (daily)	Main adverse effects
COMBINATIONS			
Rifamate (isoniazid 150 mg, rifampin 300 mg)	2 tablets	Not recommended	
Rifater (isoniazid 50 mg, rifampin 120 mg, pyrazinamide 300 mg)	≤44 kg:4 tablets 45-54 kg: 5 tablets ≥55 kg: 6 tablets	Not recommended	
SECOND-LINE DRUGS			
Capreomycin *(Capastat)*	15 mg/kg IM	15-30 mg/kg	Auditory and vestibular toxicity, renal damage
Kanamycin (*Kantrex*, and others)	15 mg/kg IM, IV	15-30 mg/kg	Auditory toxicity, renal damage
Amikacin *(Amikin)*	15 mg/kg IM, IV	15-30 mg/kg	Auditory toxicity, renal damage
Cycloserine[10] (*Seromycin*, and others)	250-500 mg bid PO	10-20 mg/kg	Psychiatric symptoms, seizures
Ethionamide *(Trecator-SC)*	250-500 mg bid PO	15-20 mg/kg	GI and hepatic toxicity, hypothyroidism
Ciprofloxacin[1] *(Cipro)*	500-750 mg bid PO	Not recommended	Nausea, abdominal pain, restlessness, confusion
Ofloxacin *(Floxin)*	300-400 mg bid or 600-800 mg/day PO	Not recommended	Nausea, abdominal pain, restlessness, confusion
Levofloxacin[1] *(Levaquin)*	500-1000 mg/day	Not recommended	Nausea, abdominal pain, restlessness, confusion
Gatifloxacin[1, 11] *(Tequin)*	400 mg/day	Not recommended	Nausea, abdominal pain, restlessness, confusion
Moxifloxacin[1,11] *(Avelox)*	400 mg/day	Not recommended	Nausea, abdominal pain, restlessness, confusion
Aminosalicylic acid (PAS; *Paser*)	4 g tid PO	150 mg/kg/d, in divided doses or 75 mg/kg bid	GI disturbance

10. Some authorities recommend pyridoxine 50 mg for every 250 mg of cycloserine to decrease the incidence of adverse neurological effects.
11. No published clinical data on dosage for tuberculosis.

DRUGS FOR NON-HIV VIRAL INFECTIONS

The drugs of choice for non-HIV viral infections with their dosages and cost are listed in the table that begins on page 84. Since the last Medical Letter issue on this subject, some new drugs and some new recommendations for old drugs have been added.

ACYCLOVIR (*Zovirax*, and others) — Intravenous (IV) acyclovir is the drug of choice for treatment of serious infections caused by herpes simplex virus (HSV) or varicella-zoster virus (VZV). Oral acyclovir is effective in treating primary HSV infections; it is less effective in treating recurrences. Long-term chronic suppression with oral acyclovir decreases the frequency of symptomatic recurrences of genital herpes and asymptomatic HSV shedding. Oral acyclovir, if begun within 24 hours after the onset of rash, decreases the severity of varicella and can also be used to treat localized or disseminated zoster.

Adverse Effects – By any route of administration, acyclovir is generally well tolerated. Gastrointestinal (GI) disturbances and headache can occur. Given IV, the drug may cause phlebitis and inflammation at sites of infusion or extravasation. IV acyclovir may also cause reversible renal dysfunction because of crystalline nephropathy; rapid infusion, dehydration, renal insufficiency and high dosage increase the risk. IV and rarely oral acyclovir have been associated with encephalopathy, including tremors, hallucinations, seizures and coma.

High doses of acyclovir cause testicular atrophy in rats, and high concentrations cause chromosomal damage *in vitro*, but no adverse effects on sperm production or cytogenetic alterations in peripheral blood lymphocytes have been detected in patients who have taken the drug orally for more than 10 years to suppress recurrent genital herpes. The manufacturer recommends stopping the drug during pregnancy, but a pregnancy registry found no unusual or excess incidence of birth defects in the offspring of more than 700 women who took acyclovir during the first trimester.

Resistance – Most acyclovir-resistant HSV isolates, which may also be resistant to penciclovir, have been recovered from immunocompromised patients treated with the drug. Resistant HSV isolates in HIV-positive patients have been associated with progressive mucosal disease and, rarely, visceral involvement. Acyclovir-resistant VZV strains in HIV-positive patients have been associated with chronic cutaneous lesions and, rarely, invasive disease. Infections with acyclovir- and penciclovir-resistant HSV or VZV may respond to foscarnet (G Breton et al, Clin Infect Dis 1998; 27:1525).

AMANTADINE (*Symmetrel,* and others) and RIMANTADINE *(Flumadine)* — Either amantadine or rimantadine is 70% to 90% effective in preventing influenza when started orally before exposure (RB Couch, N Engl J Med 2000; 343:1778). Treatment begun within 48 hours after the onset of illness decreases the duration of fever and symptoms. Whether these drugs decrease influenza-related complications or are effective in treating severe influenza pneumonia is unknown. Prophylaxis with amantadine or rimantadine has been used to control institutional influenza outbreaks and to protect high-risk patients immunized after an epidemic has begun. They can also be used as prophylaxis for immunodeficient patients, who may respond poorly to the vaccine, and in patients for whom vaccine is contraindicated because of egg allergy. Neither amantadine nor rimantadine is effective against influenza B.

Adverse Effects – Amantadine may cause anorexia, nausea, peripheral edema and, particularly in the elderly, minor central-nervous-system (CNS) effects such as nervousness, anxiety, insomnia, lethargy, difficulty concentrating, and lightheadedness. These effects usually diminish after the first week of use and rapidly disappear after the drug is stopped. Serious CNS effects (confusion, hallucinations, seizures) have occurred, especially in elderly patients and those with renal insufficiency, seizure disorders, concomitant anticholinergic drug therapy and underlying psychiatric illness. Amantadine is excreted mainly in urine and dosage must be reduced for creatinine clearance below 50 ml/min.

Rimantadine has GI adverse effects similar to those of amantadine, but a lower risk of CNS effects. It is extensively metabolized before renal excretion, so dosage reductions are not needed until the creatinine clearance falls below 10 ml/min. Both amantadine and rimantadine are teratogenic in animals and contraindicated during pregnancy.

Resistance – Influenza A viruses cross-resistant to both amantadine and rimantadine can emerge when either drug is used to treat influenza infection (JA Englund et al, Clin Infect Dis 1998; 26:1418). Viruses resistant to amantadine and rimantadine remain susceptible to oseltamivir and zanamivir.

CIDOFOVIR *(Vistide)* — IV cidofovir given once weekly for 2 weeks and then once every 2 weeks for maintenance can delay progression of CMV retinitis in patients with AIDS. IV and topical cidofovir have been reported to produce resolution of molluscum contagiosum in immunosuppressed patients (EG Davies et al, Lancet 1999; 353:2042). Cidofovir is active in animals against monkey pox virus and has activity against small pox *in vitro* (JW LeDuc and PB Jahrling, Emerg Infect Dis 2001; 7:155).

Adverse Effects – About 25% of patients have discontinued IV cidofovir because of adverse effects such as nephrotoxicity, neutropenia and metabolic acidosis. Iritis, uveitis or ocular hypotony can occur. To decrease the risk of nephrotoxicity, IV saline and oral probenecid must be given before and after each dose. Cidofovir is contraindicated in patients taking other nephrotoxic agents. Adverse effects are more common in patients simultaneously taking antiretroviral drugs. The drug is oncogenic in animals. Topical cidofovir causes local irritation and ulceration, especially in concentrations of 3% or higher.

Resistance – Ganciclovir-resistant CMV isolates may be cross-resistant to cidofovir. Acyclovir-penciclovir-resistant HSV or VZV may be susceptible to cidofovir.

FAMCICLOVIR *(Famvir)* — Famciclovir, which is rapidly converted to penciclovir after oral administration, is an alternative to acyclovir. It is effective in treating first episodes and recurrences of HSV and for chronic suppression. Administration of famciclovir to immunocompetent patients over 50 years old with herpes zoster within 72 hours after onset of rash decreases the duration of post-herpetic neuralgia, but not its incidence.

Adverse Effects – Famciclovir has been generally well tolerated. Headache, nausea and diarrhea have been reported. Like acyclovir, famciclovir has been associated with dose-related adverse effects on testicular function in animals, but not in humans. In rats, 600 mg/kg/day of famciclovir for 2 years increased the incidence of mammary adenocarcinoma.

Resistance – HSV and VZV strains resistant to acyclovir or valacyclovir have generally been cross-resistant to famciclovir, penciclovir or ganciclovir.

FOMIVIRSEN ***(Vitravene)*** — Fomivirsen, an antisense oligonucleotide, is FDA-approved for intravitreal treatment of CMV retinitis in HIV-infected patients who cannot tolerate or have not responded to other drugs. The manufacturer recommends not giving fomivirsen to patients who have been treated with cidofovir in the previous 2 to 4 weeks. The most commonly reported adverse effects include iritis, vitritis, increased intraocular pressure and vision changes. *In vivo* resistance has not been observed (CM Perry and JAB Balfour, Drugs 1999; 57:375).

FOSCARNET ***(Foscavir)*** — Foscarnet is effective in CMV retinitis, including progressive disease due to ganciclovir-resistant strains, and in acyclovir-resistant HSV or VZV infections. It is more expensive and generally less well tolerated than ganciclovir, and requires controlled infusion rates in large volumes of fluid.

Adverse Effects – Renal dysfunction often develops during treatment with foscarnet and is usually reversible, but renal failure requiring dialysis may occur. Renal toxicity is increased in patients receiving other nephrotoxic drugs such as amphotericin B (*Fungizone*, and others), aminoglycoside antibiotics or pentamidine *(Pentam 300)*; adequate hydration may decrease the risk. Nausea, vomiting, anemia, fatigue, headache, genital ulceration, CNS disturbances, hypo- and hypercalcemia, hypo- and hyperphosphatemia, hypokalemia and hypomagnesemia have also occurred. The risk of severe hypocalcemia, sometimes fatal, is increased by concurrent IV pentamidine. Foscarnet may increase the risk of zidovudine-related anemia. It causes chromosomal damage *in vitro* and *in vivo*.

Resistance – HSV, VZV and CMV strains resistant to foscarnet can emerge during treatment. Combined use of foscarnet and ganciclovir may benefit some patients, but CMV strains resistant to both ganciclovir and foscarnet have been reported.

GANCICLOVIR ***(Cytovene)*** — IV ganciclovir is used to treat CMV infections, most commonly retinitis, colitis and esophagitis, in AIDS and other immunocompromised patients and to prevent and treat CMV disease in transplant patients. An intraocular implant that releases ganciclovir (*Vitrasert* – Bausch & Lomb) has been more effective than IV ganciclovir for the eye with the implant, but is not effective in the other eye or other organs. For AIDS patients at high risk for CMV progression, combining the implant with high-dose (4.5 g/day) oral suppression decreases the risk of contralateral retinitis and extraocular CMV disease, and delays ipsilateral progression (DF Martin et al, N Engl J Med 1999; 340:1063). Oral ganciclovir alone can be used as maintenance treatment for AIDS patients with CMV retinitis, but is less effective than the IV formulation.

Oral ganciclovir or a combination of IV ganciclovir followed by high-dose oral acyclovir reduces the risk of CMV in patients who have had liver transplantation, including seronegative recipients of seropositive donations (E Gane et al, Lancet 1997; 350:1729; AD Badley et al, Transplantation 1997; 64:66); oral ganciclovir may be superior to oral acyclovir following IV ganciclovir (RH Rubin et al, Transpl Infect Dis 2000; 2:112). Oral ganciclovir alone for 3 months is superior to oral acyclovir in preventing CMV in recipients of seropositive kidney transplants (SM Flechner et al, Transplantation 1998; 66:1682).

Adverse Effects – Ganciclovir is teratogenic, carcinogenic and mutagenic and causes aspermatogenesis in animals. Granulocytopenia and thrombocytopenia are more common with the IV formulation and are usually reversible. Severe myelosuppression may occur more frequently when the drug is given concurrently with zidovudine *(Retrovir)*, azathioprine *(Imuran)*, or mycophenolate mofetil *(CellCept)*. Granulocyte-colony-stimulating factors (GM-CSF; G-CSF) have been used to treat ganciclovir-induced neutropenia. Other adverse effects of systemic ganciclovir include retinal detachment in patients with CMV retinitis, fever, rash, phlebitis, confusion, abnormal liver function, renal dysfunction, headache, GI toxicity and, rarely, psychiatric disturbances and seizures.

Resistance – Ganciclovir resistance may be associated with persistent viremia and progressive disease. Ganciclovir-resistant CMV can emerge and cause late morbidity in immunosuppressed transplant recipients given ganciclovir prophylactically (AP Limaye et al, Lancet 2000; 356:645). CMV strains resistant to ganciclovir *in vitro* may be susceptible to foscarnet or cidofovir.

INTERFERON ALFA — Interferon alfa is available as alfacon-1 *(Infergen)*, alfa-n3 *(Alferon N)*, alfa-2a *(Roferon-A)*, alfa-2b (alone *[Intron A]* and in a combination with oral ribavirin *[Rebetron]*), and pegylated alfa-2b (*PEG-Intron* – Medical Letter 2001; 43:54), and will soon be available as pegylated alfa-2a *(Pegasys)*.

In about one third of adults and children with chronic hepatitis B (HBV), treatment with interferon alfa-2b leads to loss of HBeAg, return to normal aminotransferase activity, sustained histological improvement and, in adults, a lower risk of progressive liver disease (C Niederau et al, N Engl J Med 1996; 334:1422; EM Sokal et al, Gastroenterology 1998; 114:988). AIDS patients with HBV generally respond poorly to interferon. Hepatitis D (hepatitis delta virus), which occurs only in patients infected with HBV, may respond to treatment with high doses of interferon alfa, but relapse is common.

In treatment of chronic hepatitis C (HCV), combination treatment with oral ribavirin is associated with higher response rates than with either interferon or ribavirin alone (GM Lauer and BD Walker, N Engl J Med 2001; 345:41; P Glue et al, Hepatology 2000; 32:647). Newer pegylated interferons (alfa-2a or alfa-2b) have a longer half-life, require fewer doses and are more effective than standard alfa interferon, with sustained virologic response rates (after 48 weeks' treatment) of 30%-45% at 72 weeks (S Zeuzem et al, N Engl J Med 2000; 343:1666). Pegylated interferon plus ribavirin is more effective than combination therapy with standard interferon (MP Manns et al, Lancet 2001; 358:958). In a retrospective study, use of interferon appeared to decrease the risk of hepatocellular carcinoma in patients with chronic HCV, especially among patients with sustained responses (H Yoshida et al, Ann Intern Med 1999; 131:174). In one study, interferon alfa-2b treatment of patients with acute HCV prevented most chronic infection (E Jaeckel et al, N Engl J Med 2001; 345:1452).

Adverse Effects – Intramuscular or subcutaneous injection of interferon is commonly associated with an influenza-like syndrome, especially during the first week of therapy. High-dose or chronic therapy may be limited by bone marrow suppression, profound fatigue, myalgia, weight loss, rash, cough, increased susceptibility to bacterial infections, psychiatric syndromes including depression, anxiety, emotional lability and agitation, increased aminotransferase activity, alopecia, hypo- or hyperthyroidism, tinnitus, reversible hearing loss, auto-antibody formation, retinopathy, and possibly cardiotoxicity. Injection-site reactions and dose-related neutropenia and anemia have been more common with pegylated interferon. Depression caused by interferon alfa might be treatable with an antidepressant without stopping the interferon (A Gelenberg, Biol Ther Psychiatry 2001; 24:8). Autoimmune chronic hepatitis and other autoimmune diseases like thyroiditis may be induced or exacerbated by treatment with interferon.

LAMIVUDINE (3TC; *Epivir HBV*) — This antiretroviral nucleoside analog used to treat HIV is also FDA-approved for treatment of chronic HBV infection. A trial in 334 patients with chronic HBV treated for 2 years found that 52% taking 100 mg of lamivudine daily had sustained suppression of HBV DNA and 50% had normalization of aminotransferase activity; seroconversion to anti-HBeAg occurred in 17% of patients after one year and increased to 27% after 2 years (Y-F Liaw et al, Gastroenterology 2000; 119:172). Oral lamivudine appears to reduce the risk of HBV reinfection in liver transplant recipients (L Grellier et al, Lancet 1996; 348:1212). Combination therapy with interferon alfa and lamivudine does not lead to higher response rates than monotherapy.

Adverse Effects – Lamivudine is generally well tolerated. Headache, nausea and dizziness are rare. Pancreatitis has been reported in children.

Resistance – Resistance emerges in 24% of HBV-infected patients receiving lamivudine for one year and in 42% after 2 years. Resistant variants have been associated with hepatitis flares (Y-F Liaw et al, Hepatology 1999; 30:567) and progressive liver disease in liver transplant recipients (Z Ben-Ari et al, Transplantation 1999; 68:232; C-T Bock et al, Gastroenterology 2002; 122:264).

OSELTAMIVIR ***(Tamiflu)*** — This oral neuraminidase inhibitor, started within 36 hours of symptom onset, can decrease the severity and duration of symptoms caused by either influenza A or B in both children and adults (RJ Whitley et al, Pediatr Infect Dis J 2001; 20:127; KG Nicholson et al, Lancet 2000; 355:1845). Taken once daily for prophylaxis, it appears to be effective in preventing clinical influenza (R Welliver et al, JAMA 2001; 285:748). The indications for prophylaxis with oseltamavir are the same as those for prophylaxis with amantadine.

Adverse Effects – Nausea and vomiting can occur. Taking the drug with food decreases the incidence of nausea.

PENCICLOVIR ***(Denavir)*** — Topical penciclovir 1% cream may be helpful in treating recurrent orolabial herpes simplex virus (HSV) infections in immunocompetent adults. The drug decreased the average time to healing of lesions by 0.7 days and the duration of pain by 0.6 days (SL Spruance et al, JAMA 1997; 277:1374).

RIBAVIRIN (***Virazole, Rebetol)*** — A synthetic nucleoside, ribavirin used as an aerosol *(Virazole)* may decrease morbidity in some children hospitalized with respiratory syncytial virus (RSV) bronchiolitis and pneumonia. Combination treatment of HCV with interferon alfa and oral ribavirin *(Rebetron)* has produced higher sustained response rates than interferon or ribavirin alone (Medical Letter, 2001; 43:54). Patients relapsing after interferon monotherapy may respond to the combination. IV ribavirin appears to decrease mortality in Lassa fever and in hemorrhagic fever with renal syndrome caused by hantavirus. *In vitro* ribavirin is also active against West Nile virus, but clinical data are lacking (I Jordan et al, J Infect Dis 2000; 182:1214).

Adverse Effects — Ribavirin is teratogenic and embryotoxic in animals, and is generally contraindicated in pregnancy. Pregnant women should not directly care for patients receiving ribavirin aerosol. Acute deterioration of respiratory function has been reported with ribavirin aerosol in infants and in adults with bronchospastic lung disease. Systemic ribavirin has been associated with hemolytic anemia. Oral ribavirin plus interferon appears to cause a higher incidence of cough, pruritus and rash than interferon alone.

TRIFLURIDINE ***(Viroptic)*** — Trifluridine is a nucleoside analog active against herpes viruses, including acyclovir-resistant strains. It is approved as an ophthalmic preparation for treating HSV ocular infections.

VALACYCLOVIR ***(Valtrex)*** — Valacyclovir (Medical Letter 1996; 38:3) is an L-valyl ester of acyclovir that is metabolized to acyclovir after oral administration, resulting in higher bioavailability than with acyclovir itself. Plasma acyclovir concentrations following high doses of oral valacyclovir can resemble those following IV acyclovir. In immunocompetent adults more than 50 years old with herpes zoster, valacyclovir produced more rapid resolution of zoster-associated pain and a shorter duration of post-herpetic neuralgia than acyclovir (KR Beutner et al, Antimicrob Agents Chemother 1995; 39:1546). In first-episode or recurrent genital herpes, valacyclovir twice daily is as effective as acyclovir given 5 times per day. Valacyclovir (500 mg once daily) is effective for suppression of genital HSV, but a higher dose (500 mg b.i.d.) may be needed in patients with frequent recurrences (DA Baker et al, Obstet Gynecol 1999; 94:103). Valacyclovir prophylaxis (2 g q.i.d. for 90 days) reduced the risk of CMV disease and acute graft rejection in kidney transplant recipients, including seronegative recipients from seropositive donors (D Lowance et al, N Engl J Med 1999; 340:1462).

Adverse Effects – Valacyclovir is generally well tolerated, but a thrombotic thrombocytopenic purpura/hemolytic uremic syndrome has been reported in some severely immunocompromised patients treated with high doses for prolonged periods. Hallucinations and confusion occur. Aseptic meningitis has been reported after a single 1000-mg dose in an elderly patient (MJ Fobelo et al, Ann Pharmacother 2001; 35:128). Other adverse effects have been similar to those with acyclovir.

VALGANCICLOVIR ***(Valcyte)*** — Valganciclovir, a prodrug of ganciclovir, when taken orally results in plasma levels similar to those following IV administration of ganciclovir (MD Pescovitz et al, Antimicrob Agents Chemother 2000; 44:2811). It has been similar to IV ganciclovir for induction therapy of CMV retinitis in patients with AIDS (M Curran and S Noble, Drugs 2001; 61:1145). Oral valganciclovir will probably replace ganciclovir (both oral and IV) in the treatment and maintenance therapy of CMV retinitis.

Adverse Effects – Similar to those of ganciclovir.

ZANAMIVIR ***(Relenza)*** — This orally inhaled neuraminidase inhibitor (Medical Letter 1999; 41:91) for treatment of acute uncomplicated influenza A or B in adults and adolescents, started within 2 days after onset of symptoms, can shorten the duration of illness and may decrease the incidence of some respiratory complications.

Adverse Effects – Nasal and throat discomfort can occur. Bronchospasm has been reported in patients with reactive airway disease.

DRUGS FOR TREATMENT OF VIRAL INFECTIONS

Viral infection	Recommended drugs	Adult Dosage	Cost*
Cytomegalovirus (CMV)			
Retinitis, colitis, esophagitis[1]	Ganciclovir – *Cytovene*	5 mg/kg IV q12h x 14-21d[2]	$ 741.95
		followed by 5 mg/kg IV daily	779.04[3]
		or 6 mg/kg IV 5x/wk[2]	630.65[3]
		or 1 gram PO tid[4]	1,541.58[3]
	Vitrasert implant[5]	4.5 mg intraocularly q5-8 months	5,000.00
	or Valganciclovir – *(Valcyte)*	900 mg PO bid x 21d[6]	2,417.18
		followed by 900 mg 1x/d	1,726.56[3]
	or Foscarnet – *Foscavir*	60 mg/kg IV q8h or 90 mg/kg IV q12h x 14-21d[7] followed by	2,273.15
		90 to 120 mg/kg IV daily[7, 8]	2,424.69[3]
	or Cidofovir – *Vistide*	5 mg/kg IV once/wk x 2[9] then	1,692.00
		5 mg/kg IV q2 wks[9]	1,692.00[3]
	or Fomivirsen[5] – *Vitravene*	330 µg intravitreally q2 wks x 2 then	2,000.00
		1x/mo	1,000.00[3]
Hepatitis B Virus (HBV)			
Chronic hepatitis	Lamivudine[10] – *Epivir HBV*	100 mg PO 1x/d x 1-3 yrs	1,717.32
	Interferon alfa-2b – *Intron A*	5 million units/d or 10 million units 3x/wk SC or IM x 4 mos[11]	6,819.84

* Cost for the lowest recommended dosage for a 70-kg patient, according to AWP or HCFA listings in *Drug Topics Red Book* 2001 and January 2002 *Update*. For IV drugs, the cost of administration will increase the total cost.

1. Chronic suppression is recommended in AIDS and in other highly immunocompromised patients with retinitis.
2. Dosage reduction is recommended for creatinine clearance <80 ml/min.
3. Cost of suppression for 30 days.
4. Lower doses of ganciclovir should be used to minimize leukopenia in renal transplant patients also taking azathioprine *(Imuran)* or mycophenolate mofetil *(CellCept)* (SM Flechner et al, Transplantation 1998; 66:1682).
5. Systemic therapy is recommended to prevent CMV disease in the contralateral eye and other organ systems.
6. Dosage reduction is recommended for creatinine clearance <60 ml/min.
7. Dosage reduction is recommended for creatinine clearance <1.6 ml/min/kg.
8. Over 2 hours. Higher doses (120 mg/kg/day) appear to be more effective but may be less well tolerated.
9. Not recommended for patients with serum creatinine >1.5 mg/dL, creatinine clearance <55 ml/min or proteinuria ≥100 mg/dL (2+ by dipstick). Dose reduction to 3 mg/kg is recommended for serum creatinine 0.3 to 0.4 mg/dL above baseline.
10. With monotherapy in patients also infected with HIV, HIV resistance to lamivudine emerges rapidly.
11. Pediatric dosage is 3 million units /m^2 3x/wk SC for first week, then 6 million units/m^2 (maximum 10 million units) 3x/wk for 16 to 24 weeks.

Viral infection		Recommended drugs	Adult Dosage	Cost*
Hepatitis C Virus (HCV)				
Chronic hepatitis		Pegylated interferon alfa-2b – *PEG-Intron*	1 μg/kg once/wk SC	$12,492.96
		plus Ribavirin – *Rebetol*	1000 to 1200 mg PO daily x 48 wks	16,531.20
		Interferon alfa-2b **plus** Ribavirin – *Rebetron*	3 million units 3x/wk, plus 1000-1200 mg PO daily x 48 wks	19,303.68
Acute hepatitis		Interferon alfa-2b[12] – *Intron A*	5 million units daily x 3 wks, then 3x/wk x 20 wks	5,754.24
Herpes Simplex Virus (HSV)				
Orolabial herpes in immuno-competent				
recurrence		Penciclovir – *Denavir*	1% cream applied q2h while awake x4d	24.05[13]
Genital herpes				
first episode		Acyclovir –	400 mg PO tid or 200 mg PO 5x/d x 7-10d[14]	
		generic price		14.80
		Zovirax		57.03
	or	Famciclovir[12] – *Famvir*	250 mg PO tid x 5-10d	55.13
	or	Valacyclovir – *Valtrex*	1 gram PO bid x 7-10d	79.13
recurrence		Acyclovir –	400 mg PO tid x 5d	
		generic price		10.57
		Zovirax		40.73
	or	Famciclovir – *Famvir*	125 mg PO bid x 5d[15]	33.80
	or	Valacyclovir – *Valtrex*	500 mg PO bid x 3d	21.70
chronic suppression		Acyclovir –	400 mg PO bid	
		generic price		42.29[3]
		Zovirax		162.94[3]
	or	Valacyclovir – *Valtrex*	500 mg PO 1x/d[16]	108.47[3]
	or	Famciclovir – *Famvir*	250 mg PO bid	220.50[3]

(continued)

12. Not approved by the FDA for this indication.
13. Cost based on purchase of 1.5-gram tube containing 15 mg of penciclovir.
14. For severe initial genital herpes, IV acyclovir (5 mg/kg q8h for 5 to 7 days) can be used. Dosage reduction is recommended for creatinine clearance <50 ml/min.
15. For treatment of recurrent HSV in HIV-positive patients, 500 mg PO bid for 7 days (T Schacker et al, Ann Intern Med 1998; 128:21).
16. Higher doses (1 gram) may be needed in patients with frequent recurrences.

Viral infection	Recommended drugs	Adult Dosage	Cost*
Mucocutaneous disease in immunocompromised	Acyclovir –	5 mg/kg IV q8h x 7-14d[17]	
	average generic		$ 540.57
	Zovirax	**or**	975.00
	generic price	400 mg PO 5x/d x 7-14d	24.67
	Zovirax[12]		95.05
Encephalitis	Acyclovir –	10-15 mg/kg IV q8h x 14-21d[18]	
	average generic		2,116.87
	Zovirax		3,835.00
Neonatal	Acyclovir –	20 mg/kg IV q8h x 14-21d	
	average generic		234.12[19]
	Zovirax		390.00[19]
Acyclovir-resistant	Foscarnet – *Foscavir*	40 mg/kg IV q8h x 14-21d	1,515.43
Keratoconjunctivitis	Trifluridine – *Viroptic*[20]	1 drop of 1% solution topically every 2 hours, up to 9 drops/d[21]	91.68[22]
Influenza A and B Virus			
treatment	Zanamivir – *Relenza*	10 mg bid x 5d by inhaler	48.02
or	Oseltamivir – *Tamiflu*	75 mg PO bid x 5d	63.12
prevention	Oseltamivir – *Tamiflu*	75 mg PO once/daily	265.10[23]
Influenza A Virus			
treatment	Rimantadine – *Flumadine*	200 mg PO 1x/d or 100 mg PO bid x 5d[24]	20.37
or	Amantadine –	100 mg PO bid x 5d[25]	
	generic price		1.57
	Symmetrel		12.03
prevention	Rimantadine – *Flumadine*	100 mg PO bid or 200 mg PO once[24]	171.14[23]
	Amantadine –	100 mg PO bid or	
	generic price	200 mg PO once[25]	13.20[23]
	Symmetrel		101.06[23]

17. Pediatric dosage is 250 mg/m^2 IV q8h for 7 to 14 days.
18. Pediatric dosage is 500 mg/m^2 q8h for 14 to 21 days.
19. Cost based on a 3-kg infant.
20. An ophthalmic preparation of acyclovir is available in some countries. Treatment of HSV ocular infections should be supervised by an ophthalmologist; duration of therapy and dosage depend on response.
21. Once the cornea has re-epithelialized the dose may be decreased to 1 drop q4h for 7 days.
22. Cost based on purchase of a 7.5-ml bottle.
23. Cost of prophylaxis for 6 weeks.
24. Pediatric dosage is 5 mg/kg/day up to a maximum of 150 mg/day. Dosage of 100 mg/day is recommended for older nursing home residents, for patients ≥65 years old with adverse effects from 200 mg/d, and for patients with severe hepatic dysfunction or creatinine clearance ≤10 ml/min.
25. The recommended pediatric dosage is 5 mg/kg/day up to a maximum of 150 mg/day. Dosage should be decreased in patients with diminished renal function (creatinine clearance <50 ml/min), and those over 65 years old should take 100 mg/day.

Viral infection	Recommended drugs	Adult Dosage	Cost*
Respiratory Syncytial Virus[26]			
	Ribavirin – *Virazole*	aerosol treatment 12-18 hrs/d x 3-7d[27]	1,319.85[28]
Varicella-Zoster Virus (VZV)			
Varicella	Acyclovir –	20 mg/kg (800 mg max)	
	generic price	PO qid x 5d	24.32
	Zovirax		105.61
Herpes zoster	Valacyclovir – *Valtrex*	1 gram PO tid x 7d	118.69
or	Famciclovir – *Famvir*	500 mg PO tid x 7d	154.91
or	Acyclovir –	800 mg PO 5x/d x 7-10d	
	generic price		42.56
	Zovirax		184.82
Varicella or zoster in immunocompromised	Acyclovir –	10 mg/kg IV q8h x 7d[29]	
	average generic		1,074.75
	Zovirax		1,950.00
Acyclovir-resistant	Foscarnet[12] – *Foscavir*	40 mg/kg IV q8h x 10d	1,060.80

26. Immunoprophylaxis with IV RSV immune globulin (*RespiGam* – MedImmune) or palivizumab (*Synagis*), a monoclonal antibody given by monthly injection, can prevent illness in children <24 months old with chronic lung disease and in infants who were premature (≤35 weeks gestation) (Committee on Infectious Diseases, Pediatrics 1998; 102:1211; Medical Letter 2001; 43:13).
27. Reservoir concentration of 20 mg/ml. Requires special aerosol-generating device (*Spag-2* – Viratek) and expert respiratory therapy monitoring for administration.
28. Cost of a 6-gram vial.
29. Pediatric dosage is 500 mg/m^2 q8h for 7 to 10 days.

DRUGS FOR HIV INFECTION

Since the last Medical Letter article on this subject, continuing concerns about drug toxicity and development of resistance have prompted new antiretroviral treatment guidelines (HIV/AIDS Treatment Information Service, US Dept of Health and Human Services, 2001, www.hivatis.org). The drugs of choice are listed on page 95. The dosage and cost of drugs for HIV infection are listed in the table on page 96.

NUCLEOSIDE REVERSE TRANSCRIPTASE INHIBITORS (NRTIs) — Nucleoside analogs inhibit HIV reverse transcriptase and decrease or prevent HIV replication in infected cells. All NRTIs except for didanosine are taken in 2 to 3 doses daily without regard to meals and generally do not interact with other drugs. All NRTIs can cause a potentially fatal syndrome of lactic acidosis with hepatic steatosis due to mitochondrial toxicity (G Moyle, Clin Ther 2000; 22:911).

Zidovudine (AZT, ZDV) – Zidovudine is available alone and in fixed-dose combinations with lamivudine as *Combivir* and with lamivudine and abacavir as *Trizivir*. It can be given in combination with any other NRTI except for stavudine, which causes antagonism. Zidovudine plus lamivudine with or without a protease inhibitor has been recommended for prevention of HIV infection after needlestick exposures (MMWR Morb Mortal Wkly Rep 2001; 50 RR-11:1), and has been used after sexual exposure, although data are lacking. Adverse effects of zidovudine include anemia, neutropenia, nausea, vomiting, headache, fatigue, confusion, malaise, myopathy and hepatitis.

Stavudine (d4T) – Stavudine can be given either in initial combination therapy or after failure of regimens containing other NRTIs. Cross-resistance with zidovudine is frequent, however. Fatal lactic acidosis may occur more frequently with stavudine than with other NRTIs, and has been reported in pregnant women treated with stavudine and didanosine; this combination should not be used during pregnancy. Stavudine commonly causes dose-related peripheral sensory neuropathy, which often disappears when the drug is stopped and may not recur when it is restarted at a lower dose. Serum aminotransferase activity may increase with stavudine treatment, and pancreatitis has occurred rarely, but may be more common when stavudine is combined with didanosine.

Didanosine (ddI) – Didanosine is available as buffered tablets, buffered or non-buffered powder, and non-buffered enteric-coated capsules *(Videx EC)*. The combination of didanosine and zalcitabine is not recommended because of overlapping toxicities.

Treatment-limiting toxicities of didanosine have been dose-related peripheral neuropathy, pancreatitis and gastrointestinal disturbances. The risk of both pancreatitis and neuropathy may be increased when didanosine is combined with stavudine. Didanosine buffered tablets can interfere with absorption of drugs that require gastric acidity, including dapsone, ketoconazole, delavirdine, indinavir and others; they should be taken at least 1 to 2 hours apart. Use of the enteric-coated preparation should eliminate these drug interactions. Didanosine buffered tablets must be chewed or crushed into water. Gastrointestinal tolerance may be improved by using either *Videx EC* or the buffered powder formulation, or by preparing the pediatric powder in water with a liquid antacid (final concentration 10 mg/ml).

Lamivudine (3TC) – Lamivudine is the best tolerated of the NRTIs. However, an increase in viral load early in treatment with a lamivudine-containing regimen is often an indication of resistance to the drug (DV Havlir et al, JAMA 2000; 283:229). Lamivudine-resistant strains may be cross-resistant to zalcitabine, didanosine and abacavir. Because lamivudine is also active against hepatitis B virus (HBV), HIV-positive patients with chronic HBV infection may experience a flare of hepatitis if lamivudine is withdrawn or if their HBV strain becomes resistant to the drug. Adverse effects, including mitochondrial toxicity, are uncommon; pancreatitis has been reported rarely in children.

Abacavir – Abacavir is available alone or in a fixed-dose combination with zidovudine and lamivudine *(Trizivir)*. This combination is effective for initial anti-HIV therapy, but in one study was less effective at lowering HIV RNA to undetectable levels than zidovudine/lamivudine/indinavir in the subgroup of patients with baseline plasma HIV RNA levels higher than 100,000 copies/ml (S Staszewski et al, JAMA 2001; 285:1155). HIV strains resistant to zidovudine, lamivudine and didanosine may also be resistant to abacavir. Patients with extensive prior NRTI therapy are less likely to respond to abacavir. In 5% of patients, a severe hypersensitivity reaction with fever, respiratory or gastrointestinal symptoms, malaise and rash usually develops early in treatment (median of 11 days), but can occur at any time and may be fatal. Patients should not be rechallenged. Hypersensitivity reactions have also been reported rarely when restarting abacavir after a hiatus, even in patients who previously tolerated the drug (PHJ Frissen et al, AIDS 2001; 15:289; AE Loeliger et al, AIDS 2001; 15:1325). When rash occurs without systemic symptoms associated with hypersensitivity, the drug can sometimes be continued (PG Clay et al, Ann Pharmacother 2000; 34:247).

Zalcitabine (ddC) – Zalcitabine appears to be the least effective of the nucleoside analogs and is used infrequently. Dose-related peripheral neuropathy can be severe and persistent, and is more likely in patients also taking didanosine. Other adverse effects include rash, stomatitis, esophageal ulceration and pancreatitis.

A NUCLEOTIDE REVERSE TRANSCRIPTASE INHIBITOR — Nucleotides are phosphorylated nucleosides; nucleoside and nucleotide RTIs have a similar mechanism of action.

Tenofovir disoproxil fumarate (*Viread* – Gilead) – Tenofovir DF is a pro-drug of tenofovir, a potent inhibitor of HIV replication. It was recently approved by the FDA for combination therapy in patients who have failed other regimens. Tenofovir DF is given once daily and is generally well tolerated. It appears to be effective against HIV strains that are resistant to other RTIs. The most common adverse effects have been nausea, vomiting and diarrhea. *In vitro* studies suggest that mitochondrial toxicity with fenofovir may be less than with other RTIs.

NON-NUCLEOSIDE REVERSE TRANSCRIPTASE INHIBITORS (NNRTIs) — Like the NRTIs, these drugs inhibit reverse transcriptase, but by a different mechanism. Combinations of NNRTIs with NRTIs or protease inhibitors tend to be at least additive in reducing HIV replication *in vitro*. HIV isolates resistant to NRTIs and protease inhibitors remain sensitive to NNRTIs, but cross-resistance is common within the NNRTI class. Resistance to NNRTIs develops rapidly if they are used alone or in combinations that do not completely suppress viral replication. All NNRTIs can cause rash that can sometimes be severe. NNRTIs are metabolized by and can induce or inhibit hepatic cytochrome P450 enzymes; drug interactions can occur with protease inhibitors and many other drugs (*The Medical Letter Handbook of Adverse Drug Interactions*, 2002).

Efavirenz – Efavirenz is the only NNRTI approved for once-daily dosing. One study in previously untreated patients found that 72 weeks of efavirenz/zidovudine/lamivudine was more effective than indinavir/zidovudine/lamivudine in lowering HIV RNA levels, even among patients with high baseline RNA levels (>100,000 copies/ml), and the efavirenz combination was better tolerated (S Staszewski et al, N Engl J Med 1999; 341:1865). Brief studies in treatment-experienced patients or those failing other regimens have shown that efavirenz in combination with at least two other new agents can be effective in suppressing plasma HIV RNA levels and raising CD4 counts. The most common adverse effects have been rash, dizziness, headache, insomnia and inability to concentrate. Vivid dreams, nightmares and hallucinations also occur frequently. CNS effects tend to occur between 1 and 3 hours after each dose, and often stop within a few weeks. Fetal abnormalities occurred in pregnant monkeys exposed to efavirenz; the drug should not be given to women of child-bearing age who are considering becoming pregnant. Methadone dosage often needs to be increased if efavirenz is used concurrently.

Nevirapine – Nevirapine is most effective at raising CD4 counts and lowering viral load when combined with 2 NRTIs for initial HIV therapy. It may, however, cause severe hepatotoxicity, hepatic failure and death, particularly in patients with previously elevated transaminases or underlying hepatitis B or C, and with use for post-exposure prophylaxis (E Martinez et al, AIDS 2001; 15:1261; MMWR Morb Mortal Wkly Rep 2001; 49:1153). Rash is common early in treatment with nevirapine and can be more severe than with other NNRTIs; it may progress to Stevens-Johnson syndrome. Fever, nausea and headache can also occur. To decrease the incidence of rash, nevirapine should be given 200-mg once daily for the first 2 weeks, and then 200 mg twice daily. In one study, 400 mg once daily was as effective as b.i.d. dosing (F Raffi et al, Antivir Ther 2000; 5:267). As with efavirenz, the dose of methadone often needs to be increased if nevirapine is used concurrently.

Delavirdine – A study comparing delavirdine/zidovudine/didanosine, delavirdine plus either zidovudine or didanosine, and zidovudine plus didanosine in patients with mean CD4 counts of 295 cells/mm^3 and <6 months prior HIV treatment showed only modest benefit from the triple combination (GH Friedland et al, J Acquir Immune Defic Syndr 1999; 21:281). Unlike other NNRTIs, delavirdine increases serum concentrations of protease inhibitors.

PROTEASE INHIBITORS — Protease inhibitors prevent cleavage of protein precursors essential for HIV maturation, infection of new cells and viral replication. Use of a protease inhibitor in combination with other drugs has led to marked clinical improvement and prolonged survival even in patients with advanced HIV infection. Most protease inhibitors potently suppress HIV *in vivo*. Resistance to protease inhibitors is most closely related to the number of mutations; indinavir, ritonavir and lopinavir require more mutations than other protease inhibitors to lose their effectiveness; using one or more of these drugs can sometimes be effective after failure of saquinavir or nelfinavir. All protease inhibitors can cause gastrointestinal distress, increased bleeding in hemophiliacs, hyperglycemia, insulin resistance and hyperlipidemia. They have also been associated with fat wasting, reaccumulation and redistribution. All, especially higher doses of ritonavir, can cause hepatotoxicity, which may occasionally be severe (MS Sulkowski et al, JAMA 2000; 283:74). All protease inhibitors are metabolized by hepatic cytochrome P450 enzymes; drug interactions are common and can be severe. Rifampin (*Rifadin*, and others), which decreases the plasma levels of protease inhibitors, should generally be avoided. If a rifamycin must be used, rifabutin *(Mycobutin)* is preferred (M Narita et al, Clin Infect Dis 2000; 30:779).

Saquinavir – A soft-gel preparation *(Fortovase)* with improved bioavailability and potency has largely replaced the older hard-gelatin capsule formulation *(Invirase)*, which was poorly absorbed. In one study, *Fortovase* 1600 mg b.i.d or 1200 mg t.i.d plus 2 NRTIs produced similar lowering of HIV RNA levels (C Cohen et al, Intersci Conf Antimicrob Agents Chemother 1999; 39:473, abstract 508). Aside from the large number of capsules daily, saquinavir is usually well tolerated.

Ritonavir – Ritonavir is well absorbed and at full doses potently inhibits HIV, but due to poor tolerability it is now used mainly in doses of 100 to 400 mg b.i.d. to increase the serum concentrations and decrease the dosage frequency of other protease inhibitors (A Hsu et al, Clin Pharmacokinet 1998; 35:275). Adverse reactions are common, but less likely with low doses. In addition to the adverse effects that occur with other protease inhibitors, ritonavir is more likely to cause hypertriglyceridemia, can cause circumoral and peripheral paresthesias, altered taste, nausea and vomiting, and has frequent adverse interactions with other drugs.

Indinavir – Indinavir is also a potent protease inhibitor with good oral bioavailability. Indinavir 800 mg b.i.d. combined with ritonavir 100 or 200 mg b.i.d. for ease of use was comparable in effectiveness to indinavir alone in the usual dosage of 800 mg t.i.d. (J Gerstoft et al, 8th European Conference on Clinical Aspects and Treatment of HIV Infection, Athens, Oct, 2001). In addition to adverse effects similar to those of other protease inhibitors, indinavir causes elevation of indirect bilirubin, kidney stones and renal insufficiency, dermatologic changes including alopecia, dry skin and mucous membranes, and paronychia and ingrown toenails. Patients should drink 1.5-2 liters of water daily to minimize renal adverse effects.

Nelfinavir – Nelfinavir is probably the most commonly used protease inhibitor because it is the best tolerated. Diarrhea, which may resolve with continued use, is its main adverse effect. Doses of 1250 mg b.i.d. or 750 mg t.i.d. are equally effective. In patients previously treated with NRTIs alone, the combination of two NRTIs plus both nelfinavir and efavirenz was more effective than two NRTIs plus either nelfinavir or efavirenz (MA Albrecht et al, N Engl J Med 2001; 345:398).

Amprenavir – Amprenavir is available in large capsules and in an oral solution; full doses require 16 capsules or 187 ml daily. Both preparations contain amounts of vitamin E that exceed the recommended daily allowance (RDA), so patients should be advised not to take vitamin E supplements concurrently. The most common adverse effects have been nausea, diarrhea, perioral paresthesias, vomiting and rash. Many patients with rash can continue or restart amprenavir if the rash is mild or moderate, but about 1% of patients have developed severe rashes, including Stevens-Johnson syndrome.

Lopinavir/ritonavir – Lopinavir is available in the US only in a fixed-dose combination with ritonavir (Medical Letter 2001; 43:1). The combination provides effective antiretroviral therapy when combined with other agents (RL Murphy et al, AIDS 2001; 15:F1). The usual dosage is 3 capsules b.i.d., but when used with efavirenz or nevirapine or when reduced susceptibility to lopinavir is suspected, 4 capsules b.i.d. are recommended. Lopinavir/ritonavir is useful in patients with previous HIV treatment and moderate or no protease inhibitor resistance (≤5 resistance mutations). The drug is generally well tolerated; mild diarrhea, nausea, headaches and asthenia have occurred.

USE OF ANTIRETROVIRALS IN PREGNANCY — Zidovudine alone, started at 14-34 weeks of gestation and continued in the infant for the first 6 weeks of life, reduced HIV transmission from 26% to 8% (EM Connor et al, N Engl J Med 1994; 331:1173). Now most clinicians would give zidovudine plus another NRTI and a protease inhibitor during pregnancy to prevent transmission of HIV to the offspring. Women not already on therapy should consider waiting until after 10-12 weeks of gestation to begin (JP McGowan and SS Shah, J Antimicrob Chemother 2000; 46:657). Zidovudine alone taken orally for just 3-4 weeks before delivery and during labor has been reported to decrease the risk of HIV transmission by 50% (N Shaffer et al, Lancet 1999; 353:773).

For women who are already in labor and have had no antiretroviral therapy, zidovudine given to the mother and to the infant for 6 weeks beginning within 48 hours after birth also decreases HIV transmission (NA Wade et al, N Engl J Med 1998; 339:1409). A combination of zidovudine plus lamivudine given at the onset of labor and to the infant for one week may be more effective than zidovudine alone (G Gray and PO Bertsham, 13th International Conference on AIDS, 2000, abstract LbOr5, www.iac2000.org). Single-dose nevirapine for the mother at the onset of labor and for the infant within 72 hours of delivery can also decrease the risk of perinatal transmission and was more effective than zidovudine alone given to the mother during labor and to the infant for 7 days (LA Guay et al, Lancet 1999; 354:795).

HIV REGIMENS

DRUGS OF CHOICE:

- 2 NRTIs[1] + 1 protease inhibitor[2]
- 2 NRTIs[1] + 1 NNRTI[3]
- 2 NRTIs[1] + ritonavir[4] + another protease inhibitor[4]
- Abacavir + 2 other NRTIs[1]

ALTERNATIVES:

- 1 protease inhibitor[2] + 1 NRTI + 1 NNRTI[3]
- 2 protease inhibitors[4] + 1 NRTI + 1 NNRTI[3]

1. One of the following is recommended: zidovudine + lamivudine; zidovudine + didanosine; stavudine + lamivudine; stavudine + didanosine; lamivudine + didanosine. The combination of zidovudine and zalcitabine is an alternative.
2. Nelfinavir, indinavir, saquinavir soft gel capsules, amprenavir or lopinavir/ritonavir. Full doses of ritonavir are used less frequently because of troublesome adverse effects.
3. Efavirenz is often preferred. In most patients, nevirapine causes more adverse effects. Nevirapine and delavirdine require more doses. Combinations of efavirenz or nevirapine with protease inhibitors require increasing the dosage of the protease inhibitor.
4. Ritonavir is usually given in dosage of 100 to 400 mg bid when used with another protease inhibitor. Protease inhibitors that have been combined with ritonavir 100 to 400 mg bid include, in addition to lopinavir, indinavir 400 to 800 mg bid, amprenavir 600 to 800 mg bid, saquinavir 400 to 600 mg bid and nelfinavir 500 to 750 mg bid.

DOSAGE AND COST OF DRUGS FOR HIV INFECTION

Drug	Usual oral adult dosage	Total tablets or capsules/day	Cost[1]
NUCLEOSIDE REVERSE TRANSCRIPTASE INHIBITORS (NRTIs)			
Abacavir (ABC; *Ziagen* – GlaxoSmithKline)*	300 mg bid[2]	2	$ 424.69
Didanosine (ddI; *Videx* – Bristol-Myers Squibb)*	200 mg bid[3]	2	262.30
(*Videx EC* – Bristol-Myers Squibb)	400 mg once/day[3]	1	286.57
Lamivudine (3TC; *Epivir* – GlaxoSmithKline)*	150 mg bid[4]	2	316.04
Stavudine (d4T; *Zerit* – Bristol-Myers Squibb)*	40 mg bid[5]	2	329.91
Zalcitabine (ddC; *Hivid* – Roche)	0.75 mg tid[6]	3	245.75
Zidovudine (ZDV; *Retrovir* – GlaxoSmithKline)*	200 mg tid[7]	6	369.27
	or 300 mg bid[7]	2	369.27
Zidovudine/lamivudine (*Combivir* – GlaxoSmithKline)	1 tablet bid[8]	2	685.28
Zidovudine/lamivudine/abacavir (*Trizivir* – GlaxoSmithKline)	1 tablet bid[9]	2	1,009.96
NUCLEOTIDE REVERSE TRANSCRIPTASE INHIBITOR			
Tenofovir (*Viread* – Gilead)	300 mg once/day[10]	1	$ 408.00

* Available in a liquid or oral powder formulation.

1. Cost for 30 days' treatment based on AWP listings in *First DataBank PriceAlert*, February 15, 2002.
2. Available in 300-mg tablets.
3. Some clinicians prescribe buffered tablets in doses of 400 mg once daily (RB Pollard, AIDS 2000; 14:2421). Dosage with tablets (25-, 50- 100-, 150- and 200-mg sizes): for patients <60 kg, 125 mg PO bid, ≥60 kg, 200 mg PO bid. Dosage with capsules *(Videx EC)* (125-, 200-, 250- and 400-mg sizes): for patients <60 kg, 250 mg once daily, ≥60 kg, 400 mg once daily. Dosage with powder (100-, 167- and 250-mg packets): varies from 167 mg (<60 kg) to 250 mg (≥60 kg) bid. Doses should be taken at least 30 minutes before meals or at least 2 hours afterward.
4. For patients less than 50 kg, 2 mg/kg bid. Available in 150-mg tablets.
5. For patients less than 60 kg, 30 mg bid. Available in 15-, 20-, 30- and 40-mg capsules.
6. Available in 0.375-mg and 0.75-mg tablets.
7. Available in 100-mg capsules and 300-mg tablets.
8. Each tablet contains 300 mg of zidovudine and 150 mg of lamivudine.
9. Each tablet contains 300 mg of zidovudine, 150 mg of lamivudine and 300 mg of abacavir.
10. Taken with a meal. Available in 300-mg tablets.

Drug	Usual oral adult dosage	Total tablets or capsules/day	Cost[1]
NON-NUCLEOSIDE REVERSE TRANSCRIPTASE INHIBITORS (NNRTIs)			
Delavirdine (*Rescriptor* – Pfizer)	400 mg tid[11]	6	$ 316.35
Efavirenz (EFV; *Sustiva* – Dupont)	600 mg once/day[12]	3	431.65
Nevirapine (*Viramune* – Boehringer Ingelheim)*	200 mg bid[13]	2	336.08
PROTEASE INHIBITORS			
Amprenavir (*Agenerase* – GlaxoSmithKline)*	1200 mg bid[14]	16	$ 735.54
Indinavir (*Crixivan* – Merck)	800 mg tid[15]	6	523.35
Nelfinavir (*Viracept* – Pfizer)*	750 mg tid or	9	680.99
	1250 mg bid[16]	10	756.66
Ritonavir (*Norvir* – Abbott)*	600 mg bid[17]	12	771.57
	or 100 mg bid-	2	128.59
	400 mg bid[18]	8	514.34
Saquinavir (*Invirase* – Roche)	600 mg tid[19]	9	646.95
(*Fortovase* – Roche)	1200 mg tid[20]	18	720.96
Lopinavir plus ritonavir (*Kaletra* – Abbott)*	400/100 mg bid[21]	6	703.50

11. Available in 100-mg and 200-mg tablets.
12. At bedtime for at least the first 2 to 4 weeks; may be taken with or without food, but not with a fatty meal. Marketed in 50-, 100- and 200-mg capsules.
13. 200 mg once/day for the first 2 weeks of treatment to decrease the risk of rash. Available in 200-mg tablets.
14. With or without food, but not with a fatty meal. Available in 50- and 150-mg capsules.
15. With water or other liquids, 1 hour before or 2 hours after a meal, or with a light meal. Patients should drink at least 48 ounces (1.5 L) of water daily. Available in 100-, 200-, 333- and 400-mg capsules.
16. Nelfinavir is available in 250-mg capsules and should be taken with food.
17. With food. The drug is available as a 100-mg soft-gelatin capsule. The liquid formulation has an unpleasant taste; the manufacturer suggests taking it with chocolate milk or a liquid nutritional supplement.
18. When used in combination with other protease inhibitors.
19. 200-mg hard-gelatin capsules. Only recommended for use in combination with ritonavir. Saquinavir should be taken with or within 2 hours after a full meal.
20. 200-mg soft-gelatin capsules. Saquinavir should be taken with or within 2 hours after a full meal.
21. Each capsule contains 133.3 mg of lopinavir and 33.3 mg of ritonavir. The recommended dose is 533/133 mg bid when taken with efavirenz or nevirapine, or if lopinavir resistance is suspected.

DRUGS FOR AIDS-ASSOCIATED INFECTIONS

Infection	Page
Candidiasis	112
Coccidioidomycosis	112
Cryptococcosis	112
Cryptosporidiosis	123
Cytomegalovirus (CMV)	84
Hepatitis C	85
Herpes Simplex Virus (HSV)	85
Histoplasmosis	113
Human Papillomavirus (HPV)	108
Microsporidiosis	136
Mycobacterium avium (MAC)	50
Pneumocystis carinii Pneumonia (PCP)	137
Toxoplasmic Encephalitis	140
Tuberculosis	66
Varicella-Zoster Virus (VZV)	87

Note: US Public Health Service/Centers for Disease Control and Prevention guidelines for prevention of opportunistic infections in HIV-infected patients are available at www.hivatis.org.

DRUGS FOR SEXUALLY TRANSMITTED INFECTIONS

Many infections can be transmitted during sexual contact. The text and tables that follow are limited to treatment of non-HIV infections associated primarily with sexual transmission. The US Centers for Disease Control and Prevention (CDC) publishes guidelines with more detailed recommendations for treatment of these diseases (MMWR Morb Mortal Wkly Rep, April 2002).

CHLAMYDIA AND RELATED CLINICAL SYNDROMES — A single dose of azithromycin *(Zithromax)* or 7 days' treatment with a tetracycline are both effective for treatment of uncomplicated urethral or cervical infection caused by *Chlamydia trachomatis.* Azithromycin capsules and tablets are expensive, and the capsules should be taken on an empty stomach. The single-dose powder formulation mixed with water costs less, but may cause more nausea and epigastric pain than the tablets or capsules. Taking the tablets or powder after a small snack (a few crackers or cookies) may improve gastrointestinal (GI) tolerance. Seven days' treatment with generic doxycycline or another tetracycline costs less, but compliance may be a problem. Ofloxacin *(Floxin)* or levofloxacin *(Levaquin)* for 7 days is an expensive alternative.

Nonchlamydial nongonococcal urethritis (NGU) in men, possibly caused by *Ureaplasma urealyticum, Mycoplasma genitalium* or other (unknown) pathogens, usually responds to azithromycin or doxycycline. NGU that does not resolve with azithromycin or doxycycline may respond to erythromycin or ofloxacin, or in some cases to treatment for trichomoniasis.

Mucopurulent cervicitis (MPC) has been characterized as the counterpart of NGU in men (P Nyirjesy, Curr Infect Dis Rep 2001; 3:540). As with NGU, MPC due to chlamydia generally responds to azithromycin or doxycycline.

In Pregnancy – Doxycycline, other tetracyclines and the fluoroquinolones generally should not be used in pregnancy. Amoxicillin appears to be safe and is generally effective against *C. trachomatis*. Azithromycin is probably safe and effective, but published experience with its use in pregnancy is limited (JM Miller and DH Martin, Drugs 2000; 60:597). Erythromycin usually is effective, but many patients cannot tolerate its GI effects, and erythromycin estolate is contraindicated in pregnancy.

In Infancy – Children born to women with cervical *C. trachomatis* infection are at risk for conjunctivitis and pneumonia. Neonatal gonococcal prophylaxis with ophthalmic antibiotics does not prevent ocular chlamydial infection in the newborn. For treatment of newborns with conjunctivitis or pneumonia caused by *C. trachomatis*, some clinicians have used systemic erythromycin for 14 days, but an association between hypertrophic pyloric stenosis and use of erythromycin has been reported (BE Mahon et al, J Pediatr 2001; 139:380). In one small study, a short course of oral azithromycin was effective for treatment of chlamydial conjunctivitis (MR Hammerschlag et al, Pediatr Infect Dis J 1998; 17:1049).

EPIDIDYMITIS — Acute epididymitis in men less than 35 years old is usually caused by *C. trachomatis* or, less frequently, *Neisseria gonorrhoeae*. Older men or those who have had urinary tract instrumentation may have non-sexually-transmitted epididymitis due to enteric gram-negative bacilli or *Pseudomonas*. Gram-negative bacilli may also cause urethritis or epididymitis in men who practice unprotected insertive anal intercourse. When the organism is not known, epididymitis can be treated with ofloxacin until culture results are available.

GONORRHEA — Single doses of cefixime *(Suprax)*, ciprofloxacin *(Cipro)* or ofloxacin orally, or ceftriaxone *(Rocephin)* intramuscularly (IM), are highly effective for uncomplicated anogenital or pharyngeal infection, even with penicillin- and tetracycline-resistant strains of *N. gonorrhoeae*. Other cephalosporins and fluoroquinolones may be equally effective, but have been used less and offer no clinical advantage. Fluoroquinolone-resistant strains of *N. gonorrhoeae* are prevalent in Asia, Israel and other parts of the world and are increasing in parts of the US, especially Hawaii. Fluoroquinolones should not be used to treat gonorrhea in persons who may have been infected in those areas. Spectinomycin can be used to treat pregnant women allergic to beta-lactam antibiotics, but is unreliable against pharyngeal gonococcal infection. Gonococcal ophthalmia, bacteremia, arthritis or meningitis in adults and all gonococcal infections in children are best treated with appropriate doses of a parenteral third-generation cephalosporin such as ceftriaxone.

All patients with gonorrhea should also be treated for presumptive chlamydial infection, usually with a single dose of azithromycin or seven days of doxycycline.

PELVIC INFLAMMATORY DISEASE (PID) — *C. trachomatis* or *N. gonorrhoeae* cause about two thirds of cases of acute PID, but *Mycoplasma hominis, M. genitalium* and various facultative and anaerobic bacteria may also be involved. Treatment regimens should include antimicrobial agents active against all these pathogens. Parenteral regimens include cefotetan *(Cefotan)* or cefoxitin *(Mefoxin)* plus doxycycline, clindamycin (*Cleocin*, and others) with an aminoglycoside, and either ofloxacin or levofloxacin plus metronidazole (*Flagyl*, and others); some clinicians believe ofloxacin or levofloxacin is adequate without addition of metronidazole. Parenteral therapy is continued until clinical improvement occurs, and then oral doxycycline is substituted to complete 14 days' total therapy. Recommended oral regimens are ofloxacin with or without metronidazole, or doxycycline after an initial IM dose of cefoxitin (with oral probenecid) or ceftriaxone.

VAGINAL INFECTIONS — The role of sexual transmission is important in trichomoniasis, unimportant in vulvovaginal candidiasis and unclear in bacterial vaginosis. Sulfonamide creams, other "broad-spectrum" vaginal preparations, and currently available preparations of *Lactobacillus* species or dairy products are not reliably effective for treatment or prevention of any vaginal infection. Douching is also not effective for prevention or treatment of vaginal infection, may lead to upper genital tract infection, and should be discouraged.

Trichomoniasis – Oral metronidazole is the treatment of choice for trichomoniasis. Topical treatment with metronidazole gel is not effective. A single oral dose is usually effective; treatment failures may be treated with a repeat single dose or with a longer course. Metronidazole-resistant strains of *T. vaginalis* can be treated with metronidazole 2 to 4 g/d for 7 to 14 days, or with tinidazole 500 mg q.i.d. orally plus vaginal tinidazole 500 mg b.i.d. for 14 days (JD Sobel et al, Clin Infect Dis 2001; 33:1341). Tinidazole *(Fasigyn)* is a nitro-imidazole similar to metronidazole but not marketed in the US. Metronidazole is believed to be safe during all stages of pregnancy and should be used to treat symptomatic trichomoniasis in pregnancy; such therapy does not, however, reduce the risk of preterm delivery (MA Klebanoff et al, N Engl J Med 2001; 345:487).

Bacterial vaginosis – In bacterial vaginosis, normal *Lactobacillus* species are replaced by overgrowth with *Gardnerella vaginalis, M. hominis, Mobiluncus* and various anaerobes. Oral metronidazole for 7 days is effective for treatment. Vaginal metronidazole or oral or vaginal clindamycin also are effective. Single-dose oral metronidazole has similar short-term efficacy, but is followed by a higher rate of relapse. Recurrence is common; retreatment with the same agent is usually effective.

Bacterial vaginosis has been associated with premature labor and complications of delivery, and symptomatic bacterial vaginosis in pregnancy should be treated. In controlled trials, however, treatment of asymptomatic bacterial vaginosis with oral metronidazole in pregnant women has not consistently reduced the frequency of adverse pregnancy outcomes, and vaginal clindamycin has not decreased the incidence of preterm delivery (JC Carey et al, N Engl J Med 2000; 342:534; M Kekki et al, Obstet Gynecol 2001; 97:643).

Vulvovaginal candidiasis – Many remedies are available for vulvovaginal candidiasis. One-, 3- and 7-day regimens of intravaginal miconazole (*Monistat,* and others), clotrimazole *(Gyne-Lotrimin, Mycelex)*, butoconazole *(Femstat, Gynazole)*, terconazole *(Terazol)* or tioconazole *(Vagistat)* are effective for uncomplicated vulvovaginal candidiasis (Medical Letter 2001; 43:3). A single oral dose of fluconazole *(Diflucan)* is as effective as 7 days of clotrimazole or miconazole intravaginally and is preferred by many patients, but can cause GI symptoms.

Recurrences are common after all regimens. Six-month prophylactic regimens of oral ketoconazole (*Nizoral*, and others) 100 mg daily, or oral fluconazole 150 mg once weekly, have been effective in most women with multiple culture-proven, recurrent infections. Vulvovaginal candidiasis occasionally is caused by azole-resistant *Candida glabrata*; it is unclear whether such cases are increasing in frequency (JD Sobel, Curr Infect Dis Rep 2001; 3:546).

TREATMENT OF SOME SEXUALLY TRANSMITTED INFECTIONS

Type or Stage	Drugs of Choice	Dosage	Alternatives
CHLAMYDIAL INFECTION AND RELATED CLINICAL SYNDROMES[1]			
Urethritis, cervicitis, conjunctivitis, or proctitis (except lymphogranuloma venereum)			
	Azithromycin	1 gram oral once	Ofloxacin[3] 300 mg oral bid x 7 days Levofloxacin[3] 500 mg oral once daily x 7 days
	OR Doxycycline[2,3]	100 mg oral bid x 7 days	Erythromycin[4] 500 mg oral qid x 7 days
Infection in Pregnancy			
	Amoxicillin	500 mg oral tid x 10 days	Erythromycin[4] 500 mg oral qid x 7 days
	OR Azithromycin	1 gram oral once	
Neonatal Ophthalmia or Pneumonia			
	Azithromycin	20 mg/kg oral once daily x 3 days	Erythromycin 12.5 mg/kg oral qid x 14 days[5]
Lymphogranuloma venereum			
	Doxycycline[2,3]	100 mg oral bid x 21 days	Erythromycin[4] 500 mg oral qid x 21 days
EPIDIDYMITIS	Ofloxacin	300 mg bid x 10 days	Ceftriaxone 250 mg IM once **followed by** doxycycline[2] 100 mg oral bid x 10 days

1. Related clinical syndromes include nonchlamydial nongonococcal urethritis and cervicitis.
2. Or tetracycline 500 mg oral qid.
3. Not recommended in pregnancy.
4. Erythromycin ethylsuccinate 800 mg may be substituted for erythromycin base 500 mg; erythromycin estolate is contraindicated in pregnancy.
5. Pyloric stenosis has been associated with use of erythromycin in newborns.

Type or Stage	Drugs of Choice	Dosage	Alternatives
GONORRHEA[6] — **Urethral, cervical, rectal, or pharyngeal**			
	Cefixime	400 mg oral once	Spectinomycin 2 g IM once[7]
	OR Ciprofloxacin[3,8]	500 mg oral once	
	OR Ofloxacin	400 mg oral once	
	OR Ceftriaxone	125 mg IM once	
PELVIC INFLAMMATORY DISEASE			
—parenteral	Cefotetan or cefoxitin **plus** doxycycline[3]	2 grams IV q12h 2 grams IV q6h 100 mg IV or oral q12h, until improved	Ofloxacin[3] 400 mg IV q12h or levofloxacin[3] 500 mg IV once daily **plus** metronidazole 500 mg IV q8h[9] Ampicillin/sulbactam 3g IV q6h **plus** doxycycline[3] 100 mg orally or IV q12h
	followed by doxycycline[3]	100 mg oral bid to complete 14 days	**All continued until improved, then followed by** doxycycline[3] 100 mg oral bid to complete 14 days[10]
	OR Clindamycin **plus** gentamicin	900 mg IV q8h 2 mg/kg IV once, then 1.5 mg/kg IV q8h[11], until improved	
	followed by doxycycline[3]	100 mg oral bid to complete 14 days[10]	
—oral	Ofloxacin[3]	400 mg oral bid x 14 days	
	OR Levofloxacin[3] **plus** metronidazole[9]	500 mg once daily x 14 days 500 mg oral bid x 14 days	
	OR Ceftriaxone **followed by** doxycycline[3,12]	250 mg IM once 100 mg oral bid x 14d	Cefoxitin 2 grams once plus probenecid 1 gram oral once **followed** by doxycycline[3,12] 100 mg oral bid x 14d

6. All patients should also receive a course of treatment effective for *Chlamydia*.
7. Recommended only for use during pregnancy in patients allergic to β-lactams. Not effective for pharyngeal infection.
8. Fluoroquinolones should not be used to treat gonorrhea acquired in Asia, Hawaii, Israel or other areas where fluoroquinolone-resistant strains of *N. gonorrhoeae* are common.
9. Some clinicians believe the addition of metronidazole is not required.

Type or Stage	Drugs of Choice	Dosage	Alternatives
VAGINAL INFECTION			
Trichomoniasis	Metronidazole	2 grams oral once	Metronidazole 375 mg *(Flagyl 375)* or 500 mg oral bid x 7 days
Bacterial vaginosis	Metronidazole	500 mg oral bid x 7 days	Metronidazole 2 grams oral once[13]
	OR Metronidazole gel 0.75%[14]	5 grams intravaginally once or twice daily x 5 days	Clindamycin 300 mg oral bid x 7 days
	OR Clindamycin 2% cream[14]	5 grams intravaginally qhs x 3-7 days	Clindamycin ovules[14] 100 mg intravaginally once daily x 3 days
Vulvovaginal candidiasis			
	Intravaginal butoconazole, clotrimazole, miconazole, terconazole or tioconazole[15]		
	OR Fluconazole	150 mg oral once	
SYPHILIS			
Early (Primary, secondary, or latent less than one year)			
	Penicillin G benzathine	2.4 million U IM once[16]	Doxycycline[3] 100 mg oral bid x 14 days Azithromycin[17] 2 grams oral once
Late (more than one year's duration, cardiovascular, gumma, late-latent)			
	Penicillin G benzathine	2.4 million U IM weekly x 3 weeks	Doxycycline[3] 100 mg oral bid x 4 weeks
Neurosyphilis[18]	Penicillin G	3 to 4 million U IV q4h x 10-14 days	Penicillin G procaine 2.4 million U IM daily **plus** probenecid 500 mg qid oral, both x 10-14 days Ceftriaxone 2 grams IV once daily x 10-14 days

10. Or clindamycin 450 mg oral qid to complete 14 days.
11. A single daily dose of 3 mg/kg is likely to be effective, but has not been studied in pelvic inflammatory disease.
12. Some experts would add metronidazole 500 mg bid.
13. Higher relapse rate with single dose, but useful for patients who may not comply with multiple-dose therapy.
14. In pregnancy, topical preparations have not been effective in preventing premature delivery; oral metronidazole has been effective in some studies.
15. For preparations and dosage of topical products, see Medical Letter 2001; 43:3.
16. Some experts recommend repeating this regimen after seven days, especially in patients with HIV infection.
17. Limited experience (EW Hook III et al, Sex Transm Dis, Volume 29, 2002 in press).
18. Patients allergic to penicillin should be desensitized and treated with penicillin.

Type or Stage		Drugs of Choice	Dosage	Alternatives
SYPHILIS *(continued)*				
Congenital		Penicillin G	50,000 U/kg IV q8-12h for 10-14 days	
	OR	Penicillin G procaine	50,000 U/kg IM daily for 10-14 days	
CHANCROID[19]		Azithromycin	1 gram oral once	Ciprofloxacin[3] 500 mg oral bid x 3 days
	OR	Ceftriaxone	250 mg IM once	Erythromycin[4] 500 mg oral qid x 7 days
GENITAL WARTS[20]		Trichloroacetic or bichloroacetic acid, or podophyllin[3] or liquid nitrogen	1-2/wk until resolved	Surgical removal Laser surgery Intralesional interferon
		Imiquimod 5%[3]	3x/wk x 16 wks	
		Podofilox 0.5%[3]	bid x 3 days, 4 days rest, then repeated up to 4 times	
GENITAL HERPES				
First Episode		Acyclovir	400 mg oral tid x 7-10 days	Acyclovir 200 mg oral 5x/day x 7-10 days
	OR	Famciclovir	250 mg oral tid x 7-10 days	
	OR	Valacyclovir	1 gram oral bid x 7-10 days	
Severe (hospitalized patients)				
		Acyclovir	5-10 mg/kg IV q8h x 5-7 days	
Recurrent[21]		Acyclovir	400 mg oral tid x 3-5 days[22]	
	OR	Famciclovir	125 mg oral bid x 3-5 days[22]	
	OR	Valacyclovir	500 mg oral bid x 3 days	

19. All regimens, especially single-dose ceftriaxone, are less effective in HIV-infected patients.
20. Recommendations for external genital warts. Liquid nitrogen can also be used for vaginal, urethral, and or oral warts. Podofilox or imiquimod can be used for urethral meatus warts. Trichloroacetic or bichloroacetic acid can be used for anal warts.
21. Antiviral therapy is variably effective for episodic treatment of recurrences; only effective if started early.
22. Three-day regimens of acyclovir or famciclovir are probably effective, but clinical data are lacking.

Type or Stage	Drugs of Choice	Dosage	Alternatives
Suppression of Recurrences[23]			
	Acyclovir	400 mg oral bid	
	OR Valacyclovir	500 mg-1g once daily[24]	Acyclovir 200 mg oral 2-5x/day
	OR Famciclovir	250 mg oral bid	

23. Preventive treatment should be discontinued for 1 to 2 months once a year to reassess the frequency of recurrence.
24. Use 500 mg once daily in patients with <10 recurrences per year and 500 mg bid or 1 g daily in patients with ≥ 10 recurrences per year.

SYPHILIS — Parenteral penicillin G remains the drug of choice for treating all stages of syphilis. Primary, secondary or latent syphilis known to be of less than one year's duration should be treated with an intramuscular injection of benzathine penicillin G, a repository formulation. Doxycycline is usually also effective if compliance is assured. More prolonged treatment is required for late syphilis (more than one year's duration) or neurosyphilis.

Syphilis in Pregnancy – Syphilis in pregnant women should be treated with penicillin in doses appropriate to the stage of the disease. Re-treatment in succeeding pregnancies is unnecessary in the absence of clinical or serological evidence of new or persistent infection. When pregnant women with syphilis are allergic to penicillin, the US Public Health Service recommends hospitalization, desensitization and treatment with penicillin.

Congenital Syphilis – A positive serological test for syphilis in a newborn without stigmata of syphilis may be due either to passive transfer of maternal antibodies or to prenatal infection. If there is no definite evidence of adequate treatment of the mother with penicillin during the pregnancy, Medical Letter consultants recommend prompt treatment of seroreactive infants rather than waiting 3 to 6 months to see if the antibody titer falls.

Syphilis and AIDS – Most clinicians treat HIV-infected patients with syphilis and normal CSF with standard penicillin doses for the stage of syphilis, but some patients may need higher doses or longer treatment. Even high-dose IV therapy may fail to cure neurosyphilis in HIV-infected patients; ceftriaxone for 10 days may be an effective alternative (CM Marra et al, Clin Infect Dis, 2000; 30:540).

CHANCROID — Chancroid, caused by *Haemophilus ducreyi*, is uncommon in the US, but appears here occasionally in sporadic, localized epidemics and remains a frequent cause of genital ulceration in other countries. A single dose of azithromycin or ceftriaxone is usually effective. All regimens, especially single-dose ceftriaxone, may be less effective in HIV-infected patients; single-dose azithromycin or a multiple-dose regimen of ciprofloxacin or erythromycin is preferred.

PEDICULOSIS AND SCABIES — Sexual acquisition of *Phthirus pubis* (pubic lice) is common. *Sarcoptes scabiei* infestation of the skin (scabies) can also be transmitted sexually. Topical 1% permethrin is the drug of choice for pubic lice, and 5% permethrin for scabies. Ivermectin *(Stromectol)* in a single oral dose of 200 µg/kg has been tried for resistant infections with either lice or scabies. Crusted scabies ("Norwegian scabies"), a serious complication usually seen in persons with AIDS or other immunodeficiencies, should be treated with both permethrin and ivermectin.

GENITAL WARTS AND HUMAN PAPILLOMAVIRUS (HPV) INFECTION — External genital warts are caused by human papillomavirus, usually type 6 or 11; other types (16, 18 and others) cause dysplasia and neoplasia of the cervix, anus and genital skin. No form of HPV-specific treatment has been shown to eradicate the virus or to modify the risk of cervical dysplasia or cancer, and no single treatment is uniformly effective in removing warts or preventing recurrence. Trichloroacetic acid, podophyllin, and cryotherapy with liquid nitrogen or a cryoprobe remain the most widely used treatments for external genital warts, but the response rate is only 60% to 70%, and at least 20% to 30% of responders will have a recurrence. Imiquimod 5% cream (*Aldara* – Medical Letter 1997; 39:118), an immune modulator, and podofilox 0.5% solution or gel *(Condylox)* are no more effective, but offer the advantage of self-application by patients at home. Imiquimod, podofilox and podophyllin are not recommended for use during pregnancy. Topical trichloroacetic acid, cryotherapy, electrodesiccation and electrocauterization are options and can be used in pregnancy. Scissor excision or laser therapy are effective and well-tolerated if the clinician is properly trained.

No treatment is recommended for subclinical HPV infection in the absence of dysplasia or neoplasia. The short duration of most HPV infections in young women suggests that these infections and the low-grade cervical dysplasia often associated with them should both be treated conservatively (AB Moscicki et al, JAMA 2001; 285:2995).

GENITAL HERPES — Acyclovir (*Zovirax*, and others), famciclovir *(Famvir)* or valacyclovir *(Valtrex)* taken orally shortens the duration of pain, viral shedding and systemic symptoms in initial herpes simplex virus genital infection. Most experts consider acyclovir dosage of 400 mg orally t.i.d. as effective and more convenient than the regimen recommended in the package insert (200 mg five times daily). These drugs also speed the healing of symptomatic recurrent lesions if treatment is started early. Valacyclovir is equally effective when given for episodic treatment of recurrent herpes for 3 days or 5 days. It is likely that acyclovir or famciclovir also would be effective in 3-day regimens, but have not been studied. Continuous suppressive therapy with oral acyclovir, valacyclovir or famciclovir markedly decreases symptomatic recurrences, without cumulative toxicity or apparent development of resistance in immunocompetent persons. It does not entirely eliminate asymptomatic anogenital shedding of HSV, and its effect in preventing transmission is unknown.

In pregnancy – Although acyclovir is not approved for treatment of pregnant women, its use during pregnancy has not been associated with an increased risk of congenital abnormalities, and many clinicians prescribe the drug for treatment of first episodes of genital herpes during pregnancy. Suppression of recurrent genital herpes in pregnant women near term may reduce the need for cesarean sections to avoid neonatal herpes infections.

PROPHYLAXIS FOLLOWING SEXUAL ASSAULT — Many experts recommend that sexually assaulted persons be given treatment to prevent sexually transmitted infections, including therapy for gonorrhea (cefixime, ciprofloxacin, or ceftriaxone), chlamydial infection (azithromycin or doxycycline) and bacterial vaginosis and trichomoniasis (metronidazole 2 g in a single dose). Vaccination against hepatitis B (Medical Letter 2001; 43:67) should be initiated. Some experts also recommend post-exposure prophylaxis against human immunodeficiency virus infection (such as zidovudine plus lamivudine ± a protease inhibitor) if the assailant is believed to be HIV-infected and if treatment can be started within 72 hours (see page 88).

SYSTEMIC ANTIFUNGAL DRUGS

The drugs of choice for treatment of deep fungal infections are listed in the table below. Some of the indications and dosages recommended here have not been approved by the US Food and Drug Administration.

Infection Drug of Choice	Dosage	Duration[1]	Alternatives
Aspergillosis			
Amphotericin B[2]	1-1.5 mg/kg/d IV	≥10 wks	Itraconazole 200 mg IV bid x 2d, then 200 mg IV qd x 12d or 200 mg PO tid x 3d; either followed by 200 mg PO bid
or			
Voriconazole[3]	6 mg/kg IV q12h x 1d, then 4 mg/kg IV q12h, then possibly 200 mg PO bid		Caspofungin 70 mg IV x 1d, then 50 mg IV qd
Blastomycosis[4]			
Itraconazole	200 mg PO bid	6 mos	Fluconazole 400-800 mg PO once daily
or			
Amphotericin B[2]	0.5-0.7 mg/kg/d IV[5]	6-12 wks	

(continued)

1. The optimal duration of treatment with these drugs is often unclear. Depending on the disease and its severity, they may be continued for weeks or months or, particularly in AIDS patients, indefinitely (J Sobel et al, Clin Infect Dis 2000; 30:652).
2. Amphotericin B deoxycholate is given IV in 5% dextrose over about 2 to 3 hours once daily. The usual dose of amphotericin B lipid complex *(Abelcet)* is 5 mg/kg IV once daily, given over 2 hours. The recommended dosage of amphotericin B cholesteryl sulfate *(Amphotec)* is 3 to 4 mg/kg IV, given as 1 mg/kg/hour once daily. The usual dosage of liposomal amphotericin B *(AmBisome)* is 3 to 5 mg/kg/day IV, given over 1 to 2 hours, but for treatment of cryptococcal meningitis in HIV patients, the manufacturer recommends 6 mg/kg/day, and dosages as high as 15 mg/kg/d have been used for treatment of aspergillosis (TJ Walsh et al, Antimicrob Agents Chemother 2001; 45:3487).
3. Voriconazole is a new triazole that will probably be marketed in 2002 in the US and Europe. Dosage and safety in children are not established. In one study, voriconazole was more effective than amphotericin B for treatment of invasive aspergillosis (R Herbrecht et al, Intersci Conf Antimicrob Agents Chemother 2001; 43:378, abs J-680).
4. Patients with severe illness should receive amphotericin B.
5. 0.7-1 mg/kg for immunocompromised or CNS infection.

Infection Drug of Choice	Dosage	Duration[1]	Alternatives
Candidiasis			
superficial (oropharyngeal, esophageal)[6, 7]			
Fluconazole[7] *or* Amphotericin B	200 mg once, then 100 mg once daily 0.3-0.5 mg/kg/d	1-3 wks	Itraconazole[8] 200 mg PO once daily Voriconazole[3,9] 200 mg PO bid Caspofungin 70 mg IV, then 50 mg IV qd
deep[7]			
Amphotericin B[2] *or* Fluconazole[11]	0.5-1 mg/kg/d IV[10] 400-800 mg IV or PO once daily	2 wks after afebrile and blood cultures negative	
Coccidioidomycosis[4,12]			
Itraconazole	200 mg PO bid	> 1 yr	
or Fluconazole[11]	400-800 mg PO once/d	>1 yr	
or Amphotericin B[2]	0.5-0.7 mg/kg/d IV	>1 yr	
Cryptococcosis[13]			
Amphotericin B[2] +Flucytosine	0.5-1 mg/kg/d IV[5] 100 mg/kg/d PO[14]	2 wks	
followed by Fluconazole[15]	400 mg PO once/d	8 wks	Itraconazole 200 mg PO bid

6. Azole-resistant oropharyngeal or esophageal candidiasis usually responds to amphotericin B 0.3 mg/kg IV qd. Clotrimazole troches (10 mg) five times daily or nystatin suspension 500,000 units (5 ml) four times daily can also be used.
7. *Candida krusei* infections are resistant to fluconazole. *Candida glabrata* infections are often resistant to low doses, but may be susceptible to high doses of fluconazole. *Candida lusitaniae* are usually resistant to amphotericin B.
8. For patients with oropharyngeal disease, itraconazole oral solution 200 mg (20 ml) given once daily without food is more expensive but more effective than itraconazole capsules.
9. R Ally et al, Clin Infect Dis 2001; 33:1447.
10. Bladder irrigation with 50 μg/ml of amphotericin B in sterile water has been used to treat *Candida* cystitis.
11. Non-neutropenic patients only.
12. Itraconazole is the drug of choice for non-meningeal coccidioidomycosis (JN Galgiani et al, Ann Intern Med 2000; 133:676). Fluconazole is preferred for coccidioidal meningitis. Patients with meningitis who do not respond may require intrathecal amphotericin B.
13. 4-8 weeks of amphotericin B ± flucytosine is curative in non-HIV patients.
14. Divided into 4 doses q6h. Dosage must be decreased in patients with diminished renal function. When given with amphotericin B, some Medical Letter consultants recommend beginning flucytosine at the lower dosage of 75 mg/kg/day, divided q6h, until the degree of amphotericin nephrotoxicity becomes clear or flucytosine blood levels can be determined.

Infection Drug of Choice	Dosage	Duration[1]	Alternatives
Cryptococcosis *(continued)*			
maintenance[16]			
Fluconazole	200 mg PO once/d		Amphotericin B 0.5-1 mg/kg IV weekly
Fusariosis			
Amphotericin B[2]	1-1.5 mg/kg/d IV qd		Voriconazole[3] 6 mg/kg IV q12h x 1d, then 4 mg/kg q12h
Histoplasmosis[4]			
Itraconazole	200 mg PO bid	6-18 mos	Fluconazole 400-800 mg PO once daily
or			
Amphotericin B[2]	0.5-0.7 mg/kg/d IV[5]	10-12 wks	
chronic suppression[16]			
Itraconazole	200 mg PO once daily or bid		Amphotericin B 0.5-1 mg/kg IV weekly
Mucormycosis			
Amphotericin B[2]	1-1.5 mg/kg/d IV	6-10 wks	
Paracoccidioidomycosis[4]			
Itraconazole	100-200 mg PO once daily	6-12 mos	Ketoconazole 200-400 mg PO once daily
or			
Amphotericin B[2,17]	0.4-0.5 mg/kg/d IV		
Pseudallescheriasis			
Voriconazole[3]	6 mg/kg IV q12h x 1d, then 4 mg/kg IV q12h, then 200 mg PO bid[18]		
or Itraconazole	200 mg IV bid x 2d, then IV once/d or PO tid x 3d, then PO bid		
Sporotrichosis			
cutaneous			
Itraconazole	100-200 mg PO once daily	3-6 mos	Potassium iodide 1-5 ml PO tid
extracutaneous[4]			
Amphotericin B[2]	0.5-0.7 mg/kg/d IV	12 mos	
or Itraconazole	200 mg PO bid		

15. CM van der Horst et al, N Engl J Med 1997; 337:15.
16. Suppressive for patients with HIV infection.
17. Initial treatment of severely ill patients. To be followed by itraconazole.
18. MA Nesky et al, Clin Infect Dis 2000; 31:673.

FORMULATIONS OF AMPHOTERICIN B

Trade Name	Usual IV dosage	Duration of Infusion	Cost*
Amphotericin B deoxycholate (*Fungizone*, and others)	0.5-1.5 mg/kg/day	2-3 hr	$ 37
Liposomal amphotericin B (L-AmB) *AmBisome* (Fujisawa)	3-5 mg/kg/day	1-2 hr	1,319
Amphotericin B lipid complex (ABLC) *Abelcet* (Elan Pharma)	5 mg/kg/day	2 hr	805
Amphotericin B cholesteryl sulfate complex (ABCD) *Amphotec* (Alza)	3-4 mg/kg/day	3-4 hr	448

* For one day's treatment of a 70-kg patient at the highest usual dosage, according to AWP listings in *Drug Topics Red Book Update*, January 2002. The price of amphotericin B deoxycholate is the price of *Fungizone* in *Drug Topics Red Book*, 2001.

AMPHOTERICIN B – Intravenous infusion of amphotericin B deoxycholate (*Fungizone*, and others) frequently causes fever and chills, and sometimes headache, nausea, vomiting, hypotension and tachypnea, usually beginning 1 to 3 hours after starting the infusion and lasting about 1 hour. The intensity of the acute reaction is most severe with the first few doses. Pretreatment with acetaminophen (*Tylenol*, and others) or aspirin, diphenhydramine (*Benadryl*, and others) 25 mg IV and/or hydrocortisone 25 mg IV can decrease the severity of the reaction. Treatment with meperidine (*Demerol*, and others) 25-50 mg IV can shorten the duration of fever and chills.

Nephrotoxicity is the major dose-limiting toxicity of amphotericin B deoxycholate; sodium loading with 500-1000 cc normal saline may prevent or ameliorate it and is generally recommended for patients who can tolerate a fluid load. Hypokalemia, hypomagnesemia, weight loss, malaise and anemia are common. Mild renal tubular acidosis, thrombocytopenia and mild leukopenia can occur. The nephrotoxicity of amphotericin B may add to the nephrotoxicity of cyclosporine *(Sandimmune, Neoral)*, tacrolimus *(Prograf)* and aminoglycoside antibiotics.

Lipid Formulations – Three lipid formulations of amphotericin B are marketed in the US. Amphotericin B deoxycholate, the nonlipid formulation, is the least expensive amphotericin B product, and therefore is generally the preferred agent for all indications.

There are few data comparing the efficacy of amphotericin B deoxycholate with the lipid formulations. In one study, liposomal amphotericin B was as effective as amphotericin B deoxycholate for empirical antifungal therapy in patients with fever and neutropenia (TJ Walsh et al, N Engl J Med 1999; 340:764).

Acute infusion-related reactions are worst with ABCD, less with amphotericin B deoxycholate and ABLC, and least with *AmBisome*. Nephrotoxicity is least with *AmBisome* and most with amphotericin B deoxycholate (JR Wingard et al, Clin Infect Dis 2000; 31:1155). A small study comparing 4- with 24-hour infusions of amphotericin B deoxycholate concluded that both infusion-related reactions and nephrotoxicity were less with 24-hour infusions (U Eriksson et al, BMJ 2001; 322:579). Cost comparisons of amphotericin B formulations are important, but must take into account that amphotericin B deoxycholate may predispose some patients to acute renal failure, which increases hospital stay, expense and mortality (DW Bates et al, Clin Infect Dis 2001; 32:686).

CASPOFUNGIN *(Cancidas)* — Although generally well tolerated, caspofungin occasionally causes rash, fever and mild hepatic toxicity (Medical Letter 2001; 43:58). Anaphylaxis has occurred. Dosage should be reduced in patients with moderate hepatic dysfunction. Co-administration of cyclosporine (*Sandimmune*, and others) should be avoided because of the potential for hepatotoxicity.

FLUCYTOSINE (*Ancobon)* – Potentially lethal, dose-related bone marrow toxicity, gastrointestinal discomfort and rapid development of resistance when used alone have limited use of flucytosine. Dosage should be no higher than 100 mg/kg/day and should be decreased in patients with renal failure. Keeping serum concentrations below 100 μg/ml (some clinicians recommend staying below 50 μg/ml) decreases toxicity, but delays in obtaining assay results often limit their value.

FLUCONAZOLE ***(Diflucan)*** – Fluconazole is generally well tolerated. Gastrointestinal distress and rash can occur. Stevens-Johnson syndrome, anaphylaxis and hepatic necrosis have been reported.

Interactions – Fluconazole has fewer drug interactions than itraconazole or ketoconazole because it is a weaker inhibitor of CYP3A4. It is, however, a strong inhibitor of CYP2C9 and can increase serum concentrations of cyclosporine (*Neoral,* and others), tacrolimus *(Prograf),* rifabutin *(Mycobutin),* phenytoin (*Dilantin,* and others), zidovudine *(Retrovir),* indinavir *(Crixivan),* oral anticoagulants, and oral hypoglycemic sulfonylureas such as glyburide (*DiaBeta,* and others). Concomitant administration of rifampin can lower serum concentrations of fluconazole.

ITRACONAZOLE ***(Sporanox)*** – The most common adverse effects of itraconazole are dose-related nausea and abdominal discomfort. Allergic rash and hepatitis can occur. The drug can cause hypokalemia, edema and hypertension, and worsening myocardial function has been reported in patients with cardiac disease. Thrombocytopenia and leukopenia have also been reported.

Interactions – Food increases absorption of itraconazole capsules, but decreases absorption of itraconazole oral solution. Serum concentrations with the solution taken without food appear to be higher than those with the capsules taken with food. Gastric acid increases absorption of itraconazole capsules. Concurrent use of drugs that decrease gastric acidity, such as antacids, H_2-receptor blockers, proton pump inhibitors or didanosine *(Videx),* decreases absorption of the capsules, but probably not of the solution. Rifampin *(Rifadin, Rimactane),* isoniazid *(Nydrazid),* phenytoin (*Dilantin,* others) or carbamazepine (*Tegretol,* others) taken concurrently may also decrease serum concentrations of itraconazole, probably by increasing its metabolism.

Itraconazole is a potent inhibitor of the hepatic isozyme CYP3A4. Taking it concurrently may increase serum concentrations of many other drugs that are metabolized by CYP3A4 (*The Medical Letter Handbook of Adverse Drug Interactions* 2002, page 100).

Itraconazole can also, by a different mechanism, increase serum concentrations of digoxin (*Lanoxin*, and others). Serious cardiac arrhythmias or death have been reported in patients taking itraconazole with pimozide *(Orap)* or quinidine. Possible decreased contraceptive effect has been reported in patients taking oral contraceptives with itraconazole. The protease inhibitors, ritonavir *(Norvir)*, amprenavir *(Agenerase)* or indinavir *(Crixivan)* taken with itraconazole may increase the serum concentrations of both drugs. Rhabdomyolysis has been reported in patients taking itraconazole with lovastatin *(Mevacor)* or simvastatin *(Zocor)*, and also in one patient taking itraconazole with both niacin and lovastatin. Other azole antifungals have increased plasma concentrations of loratadine *(Claritin)*, oral anticoagulants and oral hypoglycemics, suggesting that itraconazole should be used with caution in patients taking any of these drugs.

KETOCONAZOLE ***(Nizoral)*** — Anorexia, nausea and vomiting are common with higher doses (>400 mg/day of ketoconazole); taking the drug with food or at bedtime may improve tolerance. Pruritus, rash and dizziness may occur. Ketoconazole can decrease plasma testosterone concentrations and cause gynecomastia, decreased libido and loss of potency in men and menstrual irregularities in women. High doses may inhibit adrenal steroidogenesis and decrease plasma cortisol concentrations. Mild hepatic toxicity is fairly common with ketoconazole, but serious liver damage is uncommon. If jaundice or symptoms of hepatitis appear, the drug should be stopped promptly or fatal hepatic necrosis may occur.

Interactions – Drug interactions with ketoconazole are similar to those with itraconazole (*The Medical Letter Handbook of Adverse Drug Interactions*, 2002, page 100).

VORICONAZOLE ***(Vfend)*** — Transient visual disturbances, including blurred vision, photophobia and altered perception of color or image, are common with voriconazole. Rash, photosensitivity, increased transaminase activity and hallucinations have also occurred. In patients with serum creatinine above 2.5 mg/dL the drug should be given orally, not intravenously, because the solubilizing agent (sulfobutylether-β-cyclodextrin), not voriconazole itself, can accumulate.

Interactions – Voriconazole is largely metabolized in the liver by CYP2C19, which is genetically variable (about 3% to 5% of Caucasians and African-Americans and about 15% of Asians do not express it). Dosage should be halved in patients with mild or moderate hepatic cirrhosis. Because of actual or potential drug interactions, voriconazole is contraindicated, according to the manufacturer, in patients taking rifampin (*Rifadin,* and others), ergot alkaloids, long-acting barbiturates, carbamazepine (*Tegretol,* and others), pimozide *(Orap),* quinidine or sirolimus *(Rapamune).* Clinical monitoring or dose adjustment may be required in patients taking warfarin (*Coumadin,* and others), cyclosporine (*Sandimmune,* and others), sulphonylureas, statins, benzodiazepines, vinca alkaloids, efavirenz *(Sustiva),* nevirapine *(Viramune)* and HIV protease inhibitors other than indinavir. Co-administration of voriconazole with omeprazole (*Prilosec,* and others), cyclosporine or tacrolimus may require reduced doses of these drugs. Patients taking rifabutin *(Mycobutin)* or phenytoin (*Dilantin,* and others) may require increased doses of voriconazole.

PREGNANCY — Fluconazole is teratogenic in animals and a similar pattern of craniofacial and cardiac anomalies has been reported in a few infants exposed to high doses of the drug during pregnancy. Itraconazole and ketoconazole are both teratogenic in rats. None of these azoles should be used in pregnancy except for a strong clinical indication for which no suitable alternative is available. Intravenous amphotericin B deoxycholate is preferred for treatment of deep fungal infections during pregnancy (CT King et al, Clin Infect Dis 1998; 27:1151).

PROPHYLAXIS — High-risk neutropenic patients, such as those undergoing allogeneic and some autologous stem cell transplants, and some with hematologic malignancy expected to have prolonged profound neutropenia, may require prophylactic treatment with antifungal drugs (CA Diekewicz, Clin Infect Dis 2001; 33:139). The drug of choice for these patients is fluconazole 400 mg PO or

IV once daily (JH Rex et al, Clin Infect Dis 2000; 30:662). Itraconazole solution, 200 mg PO or IV once daily, is an alternative.

HIV-infected patients with frequent or severe recurrences of oral or esophageal candidiasis may also require prophylaxis. For these patients the drug of choice is fluconazole 100-200 mg PO once daily. Itraconazole solution 200 mg PO once daily is an alternative (USPHS/IDSA Prevention of Opportunistic Infections Working Group, Clin Infect Dis 2000; 30:S29). Recurrent vaginal candidiasis in any population can be controlled by fluconazole 100-150 mg PO once weekly.

EMPIRIC TREATMENT — For neutropenic patients with fever that persists despite treatment with antibacterial drugs, addition of an antifungal drug is common practice. Amphotericin B or liposomal amphotericin B have been used for this indication; liposomal amphotericin B is better tolerated, but much more expensive. In one randomized trial, voriconazole appeared to be about as effective as liposomal amphotericin B (TJ Walsh et al, N Engl J Med 2002; 346:225; JH Powers et al, N Engl J Med 2002; 346:290). Fluconazole and itraconazole have also been used as alternatives to amphotericin B for this indication (DJ Winston et al, Am J Med 2000; 108:282; M Boogaerts et al, Ann Intern Med 2001; 135:412).

DRUGS FOR PARASITIC INFECTIONS

Parasitic infections are found throughout the world. With increasing travel, immigration, use of immunosuppressive drugs and the spread of AIDS, physicians anywhere may see infections caused by previously unfamiliar parasites. The table below lists first-choice and alternative drugs for most parasitic infections. The manufacturers of the drugs are listed on page 143.

Infection	Drug	Adult dosage	Pediatric dosage
Acanthamoeba keratitis			
Drug of choice:	See footnote 1		
AMEBIASIS *(Entamoeba histolytica)*			
asymptomatic			
Drug of choice:	Iodoquinol	650 mg tid x 20d	30-40 mg/kg/d (max. 2g) in 3 doses x 20d
	OR Paromomycin	25-35 mg/kg/d in 3 doses x 7d	25-35 mg/kg/d in 3 doses x 7d
Alternative:	Diloxanide furoate[2]	500 mg tid x 10d	20 mg/kg/d in 3 doses x 10d
mild to moderate intestinal disease[3]			
Drug of choice:[4]	Metronidazole	500-750 mg tid x 7-10d	35-50 mg/kg/d in 3 doses x 7-10d
	OR Tinidazole[5]	2 grams/d divided tid x 3d	50 mg/kg (max. 2g) qd x 3d

* Availability problems. See table on page 12.

1. For treatment of keratitis caused by *Acanthamoeba*, concurrent topical use of 0.1% propamidine isethionate *(Brolene)* plus neomycin-polymyxin B-gramicidin ophthalmic solution has been successful (SL Hargrave et al, Ophthalmology 1999; 106:952). In addition, 0.02% topical polyhexamethylene biguanide (PHMB) and/or chlorhexadine has been used successfully in a large number of patients (G Tabin et al, Cornea 2001; 20:757; YS Wysenbeek et al, Cornea 2000; 19:464). PHMB is available from Leiters Park Avenue Pharmacy, San Jose, CA (800-292-6773).
2. The drug is not available commercially, but as a service can be compounded by Medical Center Pharmacy, New Haven, CT (203-688-6816) or Panorama Compounding Pharmacy 6744 Balboa Blvd, Van Nuys, CA 91406 (800-247-9767).
3. Treatment should be followed by a course of iodoquinol or paromomycin in the dosage used to treat asymptomatic amebiasis.
4. Nitazoxanide (an investigational drug in the US manufactured by Romark Laboratories, Tampa, Florida, 813-282-8544, www.romarklabs.com) 500 mg bid x 3d is also effective for treatment of amebiasis (JF Rossignol et al, J Infect Dis 2001; 184:381).

Infection	Drug	Adult dosage	Pediatric dosage
severe intestinal and extraintestinal disease[3]			
Drug of choice:	Metronidazole	750 mg tid x 7-10d	35-50 mg/kg/d in 3 doses x 7-10d
	OR Tinidazole[5]	800 mg tid x 5d	60 mg/kg/d (max. 2 g) x 5d
AMEBIC MENINGOENCEPHALITIS, PRIMARY			
Naegleria			
Drug of choice:	Amphotericin B[6,7]	1 mg/kg/d IV, uncertain duration	1 mg/kg/d IV, uncertain duration
Acanthamoeba			
Drug of choice:	See footnote 8		
Balamuthia mandrillaris			
Drug of choice:	See footnote 9		
Sappinia diploidea			
Drug of choice:	See footnote 10		
ANCYLOSTOMA caninum (Eosinophilic enterocolitis)			
Drug of choice:	Albendazole[7]	400 mg once	400 mg once
	OR Mebendazole	100 mg bid x 3d	100 mg bid x 3d
	OR Pyrantel pamoate[7]	11 mg/kg (max. 1g) x 3d	11 mg/kg (max. 1g) x 3d
	OR Endoscopic removal		

5. A nitro-imidazole similar to metronidazole, but not marketed in the US, tinidazole appears to be at least as effective as metronidazole and better tolerated. Ornidazole, a similar drug, is also used outside the US.
6. A *Naegleria* infection was treated successfully with intravenous and intrathecal use of both amphotericin B and miconazole, plus rifampin (J Seidel et al, N Engl J Med 1982; 306:346). Other reports of successful therapy are questionable.
7. An approved drug, but considered investigational for this condition by the U.S. Food and Drug Administration.
8. Strains of *Acanthamoeba* isolated from fatal granulomatous amebic encephalitis are usually susceptible *in vitro* to pentamidine, ketoconazole *(Nizoral)*, flucytosine *(Ancobon)* and (less so) to amphotericin B. Chronic *Acanthamoeba* meningitis has been successfully treated in 2 children with a combination of oral trimethoprim/sulfamethoxazole, rifampin and ketoconazole (T Singhal et al, Pediatr Infect Dis J 2001; 20:623), and in an AIDS patient with fluconazole and sulfadiazine combined with surgical resection of the CNS lesion (M Seijo Martinez et al, J Clin Microbiol 2000; 38:3892). Disseminated cutaneous infection in an immunocompromised patient has been treated successfully with IV pentamidine isethionate, topical chlorhexidine and 2% ketoconazole cream, followed by oral itraconazole *(Sporanox)* (CA Slater et al, N Engl J Med 1994; 331:85).
9. A free-living leptomyxid ameba that causes subacute to chronic granulomatous CNS disease. *In vitro* pentamidine isethionate 10 µg/ml is amebastatic (CF Denney et al, Clin Infect Dis 1997; 25:1354). One patient, according to Medical Letter consultants, was successfully treated with clarithromycin *(Biaxin)* 500 mg t.i.d., fluconazole *(Diflucan)* 400 mg once daily, sulfadiazine 1.5 g q6h and flucytosine *(Ancobon)* 1.5 g q6h.
10. A recently described free-living ameba not previously known to be pathogenic to humans. It was successfully treated with azithromycin, IV pentamidine, itraconazole and flucytosine (BB Gelman et al, JAMA 2001; 285:2450).

Infection	Drug	Adult dosage	Pediatric dosage
Ancylostoma duodenale, see HOOKWORM			
ANGIOSTRONGYLIASIS			
Angiostrongylus cantonensis			
Drug of choice:	See footnote 11		
Angiostrongylus costaricensis			
Drug of choice:	See footnote 12		
ANISAKIASIS *(Anisakis)*			
Treatment of choice:	Surgical or endoscopic removal		
ASCARIASIS (*Ascaris lumbricoides*, roundworm)			
Drug of choice:	Albendazole[7]	400 mg once	400 mg once
	OR Mebendazole	100 mg bid x 3d or 500 mg once	100 mg bid x 3d or 500 mg once
	OR Pyrantel pamoate[7]	11 mg/kg once (max. 1 gram)	11 mg/kg once (max. 1 gram)
BABESIOSIS *(Babesia microti)*			
Drugs of choice:[13]	Clindamycin[7]	1.2 grams bid IV or 600 mg tid PO x 7-10d	20-40 mg/kg/d PO in 3 doses x 7d
	plus quinine	650 mg tid PO x 7d	25 mg/kg/d PO in 3 doses x 7d
	OR Atovaquone[7]	750 mg bid x 7-10d	20 mg/kg bid x 7-10d
	plus azithromycin[7]	600 mg PO daily x 7-10d	12 mg/kg daily x 7-10d
Balamuthia mandrillaris, see AMEBIC MENINGOENCEPHALITIS, PRIMARY			

* Availability problems. See table on page 12.

11. Most patients have a self-limited course and recover completely. Analgesics, corticosteroids, and careful removal of CSF at frequent intervals can relieve symptoms (FD Pien and BC Pien, Int J Infect Dis 1999; 3:161; V Lo Re and SJ Gluckman, Clin Infect Dis 2001; 33:e112). In a recent report, mebendazole and a glucocorticosteroid appeared to shorten the course of infection (H-C Tsai et al, Am J Med 2001; 111:109). No drug is proven to be effective and some patients have worsened when given thiabendazole, albendazole, mebendazole or ivermectin.
12. Mebendazole has been used in experimental animals.
13. Exchange transfusion has been used in severely ill patients and those with high (>10%) parasitemia (JC Hatcher et al, Clin Infect Dis 2001; 32:1117). Combination therapy with atovaquone and azithromycin is as effective as clindamycin/quinine and may be better tolerated (PJ Krause et al, N Engl J Med 2000; 343:1454). Concurrent use of pentamidine and trimethoprim-sulfamethoxazole has been reported to cure an infection with *B. divergens*, the most common *Babesia* species in Europe (D Raoult et al, Ann Intern Med 1987; 107:944).

Infection	Drug	Adult dosage	Pediatric dosage
BALANTIDIASIS *(Balantidium coli)*			
Drug of choice:	Tetracycline[7,14]	500 mg qid x 10d	40 mg/kg/d (max. 2 g) in 4 doses x 10d
Alternatives:	Metronidazole[7]	750 mg tid x 5d	35-50 mg/kg/d in 3 doses x 5d
	Iodoquinol[7]	650 mg tid x 20d	40 mg/kg/d in 3 doses x 20d
BAYLISASCARIASIS *(Baylisascaris procyonis)*			
Drug of choice:	See footnote 15		
BLASTOCYSTIS *hominis* infection			
Drug of choice:	See footnote 16		
CAPILLARIASIS *(Capillaria philippinensis)*			
Drug of choice:	Mebendazole[7]	200 mg bid x 20d	200 mg bid x 20d
Alternatives:	Albendazole[7]	400 mg daily x 10d	400 mg daily x 10d
Chagas' disease, see TRYPANOSOMIASIS			
Clonorchis sinensis, see FLUKE infection			
CRYPTOSPORIDIOSIS *(Cryptosporidium)*			
Drug of choice:	See footnote 17		
CUTANEOUS LARVA MIGRANS (creeping eruption, dog and cat hookworm)			
Drug of choice:[18]	Albendazole[7]	400 mg daily x 3d	400 mg daily x 3d
	OR Ivermectin[7]	200 µg/kg daily x 1-2d	200 µg/kg daily x 1-2d
	OR Thiabendazole	Topically	Topically

14. Use of tetracyclines is contraindicated in pregnancy and in children less than 8 years old.
15. No drugs have been demonstrated to be effective. Albendazole 25 mg/kg/d x 10d started up to 3d after possible infection might prevent clinical disease and is recommended for children with known exposure (ingestion of racoon stool or contaminated soil) (MMWR Morb Mortal Wkly Rep 2002; 50:1153). Mebendazole, thiabendazole, levamisole *(Ergamisol)* and ivermectin could also be tried. Steroid therapy may be helpful, especially in eye and CNS infections. Ocular baylisascariasis has been treated successfully using laser photocoagulation therapy to destroy the intraretinal larvae.
16. Clinical significance of these organisms is controversial, but metronidazole 750 mg tid x 10d or iodoquinol 650 mg tid x 20d has been reported to be effective (DJ Stenzel and PFL Borenam, Clin Microbiol Rev 1996; 9:563). Metronidazole resistance may be common (K Haresh et al, Trop Med Int Health 1999; 4:274). Trimethoprim-sulfamethoxazole is an alternative regimen (UZ Ok et al, Am J Gastroenterol 1999; 94:3245).
17. Three days of treatment with nitazoxanide (see footnote 4) may be useful for treating cryptosporidial diarrhea in immunocompetent patients. The recommended dose in adults is 500 mg bid, in children 4-11 years old, 200 mg bid, and in children 1-3 years old, 100 mg bid (JA Rossignol et al, J Infect Dis 2001; 184:103). A small randomized, double-blind trial in symptomatic HIV-infected patients found paromomycin similar to placebo (RG Hewitt et al, Clin Infect Dis 2000; 3:1084).
18. G Albanese et al, Int J Dermatol 2001; 40:67.

Infection	Drug	Adult dosage	Pediatric dosage
CYCLOSPORA **infection**			
Drug of choice:[19]	Trimethoprim-sulfamethoxazole[7]	TMP 160 mg, SMX 800 mg bid x 7-10d	TMP 5 mg/kg, SMX 25 mg/kg bid x 7-10d
CYSTICERCOSIS, see TAPEWORM infection			
DIENTAMOEBA *fragilis* infection			
Drug of choice:	Iodoquinol	650 mg tid x 20d	30-40 mg/kg/d (max. 2g) in 3 doses x 20d
	OR Paromomycin[7]	25-35 mg/kg/d in 3 doses x 7d	25-35 mg/kg/d in 3 doses x 7d
	OR Tetracycline[7,14]	500 mg qid x 10d	40 mg/kg/d (max. 2g) in 4 doses x 10d
	OR Metronidazole	500-750 mg tid x 10d	20-40 mg/kg/d in 3 doses x 10d
Diphyllobothrium latum, see TAPEWORM infection			
DRACUNCULUS *medinensis* (guinea worm) infection			
Drug of choice:	Metronidazole[7,20]	250 mg tid x 10d	25 mg/kg/d (max. 750 mg) in 3 doses x 10d
Echinococcus, see TAPEWORM infection			
Entamoeba histolytica, see AMEBIASIS			
ENTAMOEBA *polecki* infection			
Drug of choice:	Metronidazole[7]	750 mg tid x 10d	35-50 mg/kg/d in 3 doses x 10d
ENTEROBIUS *vermicularis* (pinworm) infection			
Drug of choice:[21]	Pyrantel pamoate	11 mg/kg base once (max. 1 gram); repeat in 2 weeks	11 mg/kg base once (max. 1 gram); repeat in 2 weeks
	OR Mebendazole	100 mg once; repeat in 2 weeks	100 mg once; repeat in 2 weeks
	OR Albendazole[7]	400 mg once; repeat in 2 weeks	400 mg once; repeat in 2 weeks

* Availability problems. See table on page 12.

19. HIV infected patients may need higher dosage and long-term maintenance. In cases of cotrimoxazole intolerance, ciprofloxacin 500 mg bid x 7d has been effective (R-I Verdier et al, Ann Intern Med 2000; 132:885).
20. Not curative, but decreases inflammation and facilitates removing the worm. Mebendazole 400-800 mg/d for 6d has been reported to kill the worm directly.
21. Since all family members are usually infected, treatment of the entire household is recommended.

Infection	Drug	Adult dosage	Pediatric dosage
Fasciola hepatica, see FLUKE infection			
FILARIASIS[22]			
Wuchereria bancrofti, Brugia malayi, Brugia timori			
Drug of choice:[23,24]	Diethylcarbamazine[25]*	Day 1: 50 mg, p.c. Day 2: 50 mg tid Day 3: 100 mg tid Days 4 through 14: 6 mg/kg/d in 3 doses	Day 1: 1 mg/kg p.c. Day 2: 1 mg/kg tid Day 3: 1-2 mg/kg tid Days 4 through 14: 6 mg/kg/d in 3 doses
Loa loa			
Drug of choice:[24,26]	Diethylcarbamazine[25]*	Day 1: 50 mg p.c. Day 2: 50 mg tid Day 3: 100 mg tid Days 4 through 21: 9 mg/kg/d in 3 doses	Day 1: 1 mg/kg p.c. Day 2: 1 mg/kg tid Day 3: 1-2 mg/kg tid Days 4 through 21: 9 mg/kg/d in 3 doses
Mansonella ozzardi			
Drug of choice:[24]	See footnote 27		
Mansonella perstans			
Drug of choice:[24]	Mebendazole[7]	100 mg bid x 30d	100 mg bid x 30d
	OR Albendazole[7]	400 mg bid x 10d	400 mg bid x 10d

22. Endosymbiotic *Wolbachia* bacteria may have a role in filarial development and host response, and may represent a new target for therapy (HF Cross et al, Lancet 2001; 358:1873). Doxycycline 100 mg daily x 6 weeks has eradicated *Wolbachia* and led to sterility of adult worms in onchocerciasis (A Hoerauf et al, Lancet 2000; 355:1241).
23. Most symptoms caused by the adult worm. Single-dose combination of albendazole (400 mg) with either ivermectin (200 µg/kg) or diethylcarbamazine (6 mg/kg) is effective for reduction or suppression of *W. bancrofti* microfilaremia (MM Ismail et al, Trans R Soc Trop Med Hyg 2001; 95:332; TB Nutman, Curr Opin Infect Dis 2001; 14:539).
24. Antihistamines or corticosteroids may be required to decrease allergic reactions due to disintegration of microfilariae in treatment of filarial infections, especially those caused by *Loa loa.*
25. In heavy infections with *Loa loa,* rapid killing of microfilariae can provoke an encephalopathy. Apheresis has been reported to be effective in lowering microfilarial counts in patients heavily infected with *Loa loa* (EA Ottesen, Infect Dis Clin North Am 1993; 7:619). Albendazole or ivermectin have also been used to reduce microfilaremia; albendazole is preferred because of its slower onset of action (AD Klion et al, J Infect Dis 1993; 168:202; M Kombila et al, Am J Trop Med Hyg 1998; 58:458). Albendazole may be useful for treatment of loiasis when diethylcarbamazine is ineffective or cannot be used but repeated courses may be necessary (AD Klion et al, Clin Infect Dis 1999; 29:680). Diethylcarbamazine, 300 mg once weekly, has been recommended for prevention of loiasis (TB Nutman et al, N Engl J Med 1988; 319:752).
26. For patients with no microfilariae in the blood, full doses can be given from day one.
27. Diethylcarbamazine has no effect. Ivermectin, 200 µg/kg once, has been effective.

Infection	Drug	Adult dosage	Pediatric dosage
FILARIASIS *(continued)*			
Mansonella streptocerca			
Drug of choice:[24,28]	Diethylcarbamazine*	6 mg/kg/d x 14d	6 mg/kg/d x 14d
	Ivermectin[7]	150 µg/kg once	150 µg/kg once
Tropical Pulmonary Eosinophilia (TPE)			
Drug of choice:	Diethylcarbamazine*	6 mg/kg/d in 3 doses x 21d	6 mg/kg/d in 3 doses x 21d
Onchocerca volvulus (River blindness)			
Drug of choice:	Ivermectin[29]	150 µg/kg once, repeated every 6 to 12 months until asymptomatic	150 µg/kg once, repeated every 6 to 12 months until asymptomatic
FLUKE, hermaphroditic, infection			
Clonorchis sinensis **(Chinese liver fluke)**			
Drug of choice:	Praziquantel	75 mg/kg/d in 3 doses x 1d	75 mg/kg/d in 3 doses x 1d
OR	Albendazole[7]	10 mg/kg x 7d	10 mg/kg x 7d
Fasciola hepatica **(sheep liver fluke)**			
Drug of choice:[30]	Triclabendazole*	10 mg/kg once	10 mg/kg once
Alternative:	Bithionol*	30-50 mg/kg on alternate days x 10-15 doses	30-50 mg/kg on alternate days x 10-15 doses
Fasciolopsis buski, Heterophyes heterophyes, Metagonimus yokogawai **(intestinal flukes)**			
Drug of choice:	Praziquantel[7]	75 mg/kg/d in 3 doses x 1d	75 mg/kg/d in 3 doses x 1d
Metorchis conjunctus **(North American liver fluke)**[31]			
Drug of choice:	Praziquantel[7]	75 mg/kg/d in 3 doses x 1d	75 mg/kg/d in 3 doses x 1d
Nanophyetus salmincola			
Drug of choice:	Praziquantel[7]	60 mg/kg/d in 3 doses x 1d	60 mg/kg/d in 3 doses x 1d
Opisthorchis viverrini **(Southeast Asian liver fluke)**			
Drug of choice:	Praziquantel	75 mg/kg/d in 3 doses x 1d	75 mg/kg/d in 3 doses x 1d

* Availability problems. See table on page 12.

28. Diethylcarbamazine is potentially curative due to activity against both adult worms and microfilariae. Ivermectin is only active against microfilariae.
29. Annual treatment with ivermectin 150 µg/kg can prevent blindness due to ocular onchocerciasis (D Mabey et al, Ophthalmology 1996; 103:1001).
30. Unlike infections with other flukes, *Fasciola hepatica* infections may not respond to praziquantel. Triclabendazole, a veterinary fasciolide, may be safe and effective but data are limited (CS Graham et al, Clin Infect Dis 2001; 33:1). It is available from Victoria Pharmacy, Zurich, Switzerland, 41-1-211-24-32. It should be given with food for better absorption.
31. JD MacLean et al, Lancet 1996; 347:154.

Infection	Drug	Adult dosage	Pediatric dosage
***Paragonimus westermani* (lung fluke)**			
Drug of choice:	Praziquantel[7]	75 mg/kg/d in 3 doses x 2d	75 mg/kg/d in 3 doses x 2d
Alternative:[32]	Bithionol*	30-50 mg/kg on alternate days x 10-15 doses	30-50 mg/kg on alternate days x 10-15 doses
GIARDIASIS (*Giardia lamblia*)			
Drug of choice:	Metronidazole[7]	250 mg tid x 5d	15 mg/kg/d in 3 doses x 5d
Alternatives:[33]	Quinacrine[2]	100 mg tid x 5d (max. 300 mg/d)	2 mg/kg tid x 5d (max. 300 mg/d)
	Tinidazole[5]	2 grams once	50 mg/kg once (max. 2 g)
	Furazolidone	100 mg qid x 7-10d	6 mg/kg/d in 4 doses x 7-10d
	Paromomycin[7,34]	25-35 mg/kg/d in 3 doses x 7d	25-35 mg/kg/d in 3 doses x 7d
GNATHOSTOMIASIS (*Gnathostoma spinigerum*)			
Treatment of choice:[35]	Albendazole[7]	400 mg bid x 21d	400 mg bid x 21d
	OR Ivermectin[7]	200 µg/kg/d x 2d	200 µg/kg/d x 2d
	OR Surgical removal		
GONGYLONEMIASIS (*Gongylonema sp.*)			
Treatment of choice:	Surgical removal		
	OR Albendazole[7, 36]	10 mg/kg/d x 3 d	10 mg/kg/d x 3 d

32. Triclabendazole may be effective in a dosage of 5 mg/kg once daily for 3 days or 10 mg/kg twice in one day (M Calvopiña et al, Trans R Soc Trop Med Hyg 1998; 92:566). See footnote 30.
33. In one study, nitazoxanide (see footnote 4) was as effective as metronidazole and has been used successfully in high doses to treat a case of *Giardia* resistant to metronidazole and albendazole (JJ Ortiz et al, Aliment Pharmacol Ther 2001; 15:1409; P Abboud et al, Clin Infect Dis 2001; 32:1792). Albendazole 400 mg daily x 5d may be effective (A Hall and Q Nahar, Trans R Soc Trop Med Hyg 1993; 87:84; AK Dutta et al, Indian J Pediatr 1994; 61:689). Bacitracin zinc or bacitracin 120,000 U bid for 10 days may also be effective (BJ Andrews et al, Am J Trop Med Hyg 1995; 52:318). Combination treatment with standard doses of metronidazole and quinacrine given for 3 weeks has been effective for a small number of refractory infections (TE Nash et al, Clin Infect Dis 2001; 33:22).
34. Not absorbed; may be useful for treatment of giardiasis in pregnancy.
35. F Chappuis et al, Clin Infect Dis 2001; 33:e17; P Nontasut et al, Southeast Asian J Trop Med Public Health 2000; 31:374.
36. One patient has been successfully treated with albendazole (ML Eberhard and C Busillo, Am J Trop Med Hyg 1999; 61:51).

Infection	Drug	Adult dosage	Pediatric dosage
HOOKWORM infection *(Ancylostoma duodenale, Necator americanus)*			
Drug of choice:	Albendazole[7]	400 mg once	400 mg once
	OR Mebendazole	100 mg bid x 3d or 500 mg once	100 mg bid x 3d or 500 mg once
	OR Pyrantel pamoate[7]	11 mg/kg (max. 1g) x 3d	11 mg/kg (max. 1g) x 3d
Hydatid cyst, see TAPEWORM infection			
Hymenolepis nana, see TAPEWORM infection			
ISOSPORIASIS *(Isospora belli)*			
Drug of choice:[37]	Trimethoprim-sulfamethoxazole[7]	160 mg TMP, 800 mg SMX bid x 10d	TMP 5 mg/kg, SMX 25 mg/kg bid x 10d
LEISHMANIASIS[38]			
Drug of choice:[39]	Sodium stibogluconate*	20 mg Sb/kg/d IV or IM x 20-28d[40]	20 mg Sb/kg/d IV or IM x 20-28d[40]
	OR Meglumine antimonate*	20 mg Sb/kg/d IV or IM x 20-27d[40]	20 mg Sb/kg/d IV or IM x 20-28d[40]
	OR Amphotericin B[7]	0.5 to 1 mg/kg IV daily or every 2d for up to 8 wks	0.5 to 1 mg/kg IV daily or every 2d for up to 8 wks
	OR Liposomal Amphotericin B[41]	3 mg/kg/d (days 1-5) and 3 mg/kg/d days 14, 21[42]	3 mg/kg/d (days 1-5) and 3 mg/kg/d days 14, 21[42]
Alternatives:	Pentamidine	2-4 mg/kg daily or every 2d IV or IM for up to 15 doses[43]	2-4 mg/kg daily or every 2d IV or IM for up to 15 doses[43]
	OR Paromomycin[44]*	Topically 2x/d x 10-20d	

* Availability problems. See table on page 12.

37. Immunosuppressed patients: TMP/SMX qid x 10d followed by bid x 3 weeks. In sulfonamide-sensitive patients, pyrimethamine 50-75 mg daily in divided doses has been effective. HIV-infected patients may need long-term maintenance. Ciprofloxacin 500 mg bid x 7d has also been effective (R-I Verdier et al, Ann Intern Med 2000; 132:885).
38. Treatment dosage and duration vary based on the disease symptoms, host immune status, species, and the area of the world where infection was acquired. Cutaneous infection is due to *L. mexicana, L. tropica, L. major, L. braziliensis*; mucocutaneous is mostly due to *L. braziliensis*, and visceral is due to *L. donovani* (Kala-azar), *L. infantum, L. chagasi*. Dosage range listed includes many, but not all possibilities.
39. For treatment of kala-azar, oral miltefosine 100 mg daily for 4 weeks was 97% effective after 6 months in one study. Gastrointestinal adverse effects are common and the drug is contraindicated in pregnancy (TK Jha et al, N Engl J Med 1999; 341:1795). In an uncontrolled trial, oral miltefosine was effective for the treatment of American cutaneous leishmaniasis at a dosage of about 2.25 mg/kg/day for 3-4 wks. "Motion sickness" was the most frequent adverse effect (J Soto et al, Clin Infect Dis 2001; 33:e57).

Infection		Drug	Adult dosage	Pediatric dosage
LICE infestation *(Pediculus humanus, P. capitis, Phthirus pubis)*[45]				
Drug of choice:		1% Permethrin[46]	Topically	Topically
	OR	0.5% Malathion[47]	Topically	Topically
Alternative:		Pyrethrins with piperonyl butoxide[46]	Topically	Topically
	OR	Ivermectin[7, 48]	200 μg/kg once	200 μg/kg once
Loa loa, see FILARIASIS				

40. May be repeated or continued. A longer duration may be needed for some forms of visceral leishmaniasis (BL Herwaldt, Lancet 1999; 354:1191).
41. Three preparations of lipid-encapsulated amphotericin B have been used for treatment of visceral leishmaniasis. Largely based on clinical trials in patients infected with *L. infantum,* the FDA approved liposomal amphotericin B *(AmBisome)* for treatment of visceral leishmaniasis (A Meyerhoff, Clin Infect Dis 1999; 28:42; JD Berman, Clin Infect Dis 1999; 28:49). Amphotericin B lipid complex *(Abelcet)* and amphotericin B cholesteryl sulfate *(Amphotec)* have also been used with good results. Limited data in a few patients suggest that liposomal amphotericin B may also be effective for mucocutaneous disease (VS Amato et al, J Antimicrob Chemother 2000; 46:341; RNR Sampaio and PD Marsden, Trans R Soc Trop Med Hyg 1997; 91:77). Some studies indicate that *L. donovani* resistant to pentavalent antimonial agents may respond to lipid-encapsulated amphotericin B (S Sundar et al, Ann Trop Med Parasitol 1998; 92:755).
42. The dose for immunocompromised patients with HIV is 4 mg/kg/d (days 1-5) and 4 mg/kg/d on days 10,17,24,31,38. The relapse rate is high, suggesting that maintenance therapy may be indicated.
43. For *L. donovani*: 4 mg/kg once/day x 15 doses; for cutaneous disease: 2 mg/kg once/day x 7 or 3 mg/kg once/day x 4 doses.
44. Topical paromomycin can only be used in geographic regions where cutaneous leishmaniasis species have low potential for mucosal spread. A formulation of 15% paromomycin and 12% methylbenzethonium chloride *(Leshcutan)* in soft white paraffin for topical use, has been reported to be effective in some patients against cutaneous leishmaniasis due to *L. major* (O Ozgoztasi and I Baydar, Int J Dermatol 1997; 36:61; BA Arana et al, Am J Trop Med Hyg 2001; 65:466).
45. For infestation of eyelashes with crab lice, use petrolatum. For pubic lice, treat with 5% permethrin or ivermectin as for scabies (see page 9).
46. A second application is recommended one week later to kill hatching progeny. Some lice are resistant to pyrethrins and permethrin (RJ Pollack, Arch Pediatr Adolesc Med 1999; 153:969).
47. RJ Roberts et al, Lancet 2000; 356:540.
48. Ivermectin is effective against adult lice but has no effect on nits (TA Bell, Pediatr Infect Dis J 1998; 17:923).

Infection	Drug	Adult dosage	Pediatric dosage
MALARIA, Treatment of (*Plasmodium falciparum, P. ovale, P. vivax,* and *P. malariae*)			
Chloroquine-resistant *P. falciparum*[49]			
ORAL			
Drugs of choice:	Quinine sulfate	650 mg q8h x 3-7d[50]	25mg/kg/d in 3 doses x 3-7d[50]
	plus doxycycline[7,14]	100 mg bid x 7d	30 mg/kg/d x 7d
	or plus tetracycline[7,14]	250 mg qid x 7d	6.25 mg/kg qid x 7d
	or plus pyrimethamine-sulfadoxine[51]	3 tablets at once on last day of quinine	<1 yr: ¼ tablet 1-3 yrs: ½ tablet 4-8 yrs: 1 tablet 9-14 yrs: 2 tablets
	or plus clindamycin[7,52]	900 mg tid x 5d	20-40 mg/kg/d in 3 doses x 5d
OR	Atovaquone/ proguanil[53]	2 adult tablets bid x 3d	11-20 kg: 1 adult tablet/day x 3d 21-30 kg: 2 adult tablets/day x 3d 31-40 kg: 3 adult tablets/day x 3d >40 kg: 2 adult tablets bid x 3d

* Availability problems. See table on page 12.

49. Chloroquine-resistant *P. falciparum* occur in all malarious areas except Central America west of the Panama Canal Zone, Mexico, Haiti, the Dominican Republic, and most of the Middle East (chloroquine resistance has been reported in Yemen, Oman, Saudi Arabia and Iran).
50. In Southeast Asia, relative resistance to quinine has increased and the treatment should be continued for 7 days.
51. *Fansidar* tablets contain 25 mg of pyrimethamine and 500 mg of sulfadoxine. Resistance to pyrimethamine-sulfadoxine has been reported from Southeast Asia, the Amazon basin, sub-Saharan Africa, Bangladesh and Oceania.
52. For use in pregnancy.
53. Atovaquone plus proguanil is available as a fixed-dose combination tablet: adult tablets (250 mg atovaquone/100 mg proguanil, *Malarone)* and pediatric tablets (62.5 mg atovaquone/25 mg proguanil, *Malarone Pediatric*). To enhance absorption, it should be taken within 45 minutes after eating (S Looareesuwan et al, Am J Trop Med Hyg 1999; 60:533). Although approved for once daily dosing, to decrease nausea and vomiting the dose for treatment is usually divided in two.

Infection	Drug	Adult dosage	Pediatric dosage
Alternatives:[54]	Mefloquine[55, 56]	750 mg followed by 500 mg 12 hrs later	<45 kg: 15 mg/kg PO followed by 10 mg/kg PO 8-12 hours later
	Halofantrine[57]*	500 mg q6h x 3 doses; repeat in 1 week[58]	<40 kg: 8 mg/kg q6h x 3 doses; repeat in 1 week[58]
	OR Artesunate[59]*	4 mg/kg/d x 3d	
	plus mefloquine[55, 56]	750 mg followed by 500 mg 12 hrs later	15 mg/kg followed 8-12 hrs later by 10 mg/kg
Chloroquine-resistant *P. vivax*[60]			
Drug of choice:	Quinine sulfate	650 mg q8h x 3-7d[50]	25 mg/kg/d in 3 doses x 3-7d[50]
	plus doxycycline[7,14]	100 mg bid x 7d	2 mg/kg/d x 7d
	OR Mefloquine[55,56]	750 mg followed by 500 mg 12 hr later	15 mg/kg followed 8-12 hrs later by 10 mg/kg

54. For treatment of multiple-drug-resistant *P. falciparum* in Southeast Asia, especially Thailand, where resistance to mefloquine and halofantrine is frequent, a 7-day course of quinine and tetracycline is recommended (G Watt et al, Am J Trop Med Hyg 1992; 47:108). Artesunate plus mefloquine (C Luxemburger et al, Trans R Soc Trop Med Hyg 1994; 88:213), artemether plus mefloquine (J Karbwang et al, Trans R Soc Trop Med Hyg 1995; 89:296), mefloquine plus doxycycline or atovaquone/proguanil may also be used to treat multiple-drug-resistant *P. falciparum*.
55. At this dosage, adverse effects including nausea, vomiting, diarrhea, dizziness, disturbed sense of balance, toxic psychosis and seizures can occur. Mefloquine is teratogenic in animals and should not be used for treatment of malaria in pregnancy. It should not be given together with quinine, quinidine or halofantrine, and caution is required in using quinine, quinidine or halofantrine to treat patients with malaria who have taken mefloquine for prophylaxis. The pediatric dosage has not been approved by the FDA. Resistance to mefloquine has been reported in some areas, such as the Thailand-Myanmar and -Cambodia borders and in the Amazon basin, where 25 mg/kg should be used.
56. In the US, a 250-mg tablet of mefloquine contains 228 mg mefloquine base. Outside the US, each 275-mg tablet contains 250 mg base.

Infection	Drug	Adult dosage	Pediatric dosage
MALARIA, Treatment of *(continued)*			
Alternatives:	Halofantrine[57, 61]*	500 mg q6h x 3 doses	8 mg/kg q6h x 3 doses
	Chloroquine	25 mg base/kg in 3 doses over 48 hrs	
	plus primaquine[62]	2.5 mg base/kg in 3 doses over 48 hrs	
All *Plasmodium* except Chloroquine-resistant *P. falciparum*[49] and Chloroquine-resistant *P. vivax*[60]			
ORAL			
Drug of choice:	Chloroquine phosphate[63]	1 gram (600 mg base), then 500 mg (300 mg base) 6 hrs later, then 500 mg (300 mg base) at 24 and 48 hrs	10 mg base/kg (max. 600 mg base), then 5 mg base/kg 6 hrs later, then 5 mg base/kg at 24 and 48 hrs

* Availability problems. See table on page 12.

57. May be effective in multiple-drug-resistant *P. falciparum* malaria, but treatment failures and resistance have been reported, and the drug has caused lengthening of the PR and QTc intervals and fatal cardiac arrhythmias. It should not be used for patients with cardiac conduction defects or with other drugs that may affect the QT interval, such as quinine, quinidine and mefloquine. Cardiac monitoring is recommended. Variability in absorption is a problem; halofantrine should not be taken one hour before to two hours after meals because food increases its absorption. It should not be used in pregnancy.
58. A single 250-mg dose can be used for repeat treatment in mild to moderate infections (JE Touze et al, Lancet 1997; 349:255).
59. K Na-Bangchang, Trop Med Int Health 1999; 4:602.
60. *P. vivax* with decreased susceptibility to chloroquine is a significant problem in Papua-New Guinea and Indonesia. There are also a few reports of resistance from Myanmar, India, Thailand, the Solomon Islands, Vanuatu, Guyana, Brazil, Colombia and Peru.
61. JK Baird el al, J Infect Dis 1995; 171:1678.
62. Primaquine phosphate can cause hemolytic anemia, especially in patients whose red cells are deficient in glucose-6-phosphate dehydrogenase. This deficiency is most common in African, Asian and Mediterranean peoples. Patients should be screened for G-6-PD deficiency before treatment. Primaquine should not be used during pregnancy.
63. If chloroquine phosphate is not available, hydroxychloroquine sulfate is as effective; 400 mg of hydroxychloroquine sulfate is equivalent to 500 mg of chloroquine phosphate.

Infection	Drug	Adult dosage	Pediatric dosage
All *Plasmodium*			
PARENTERAL			
Drug of choice:[64]	Quinidine gluconate[65]	10 mg/kg loading dose (max. 600 mg) in normal saline slowly over 1 to 2 hrs, followed by continuous infusion of 0.02 mg/kg/min until oral therapy can be started	Same as adult dose
	OR Quinine dihydrochloride[65]	20 mg/kg loading dose IV in 5% dextrose over 4 hrs, followed by 10 mg/kg over 2-4 hrs q8h (max. 1800 mg/d) until oral therapy can be started	Same as adult dose
Alternative:	Artemether[66]*	3.2 mg/kg IM, then 1.6 mg/kg daily x 5-7d	Same as adult dose
Prevention of relapses: *P. vivax* and *P. ovale* only			
Drug of choice:	Primaquine phosphate[62,67]	26.3 mg (15 mg base)/d x 14d or 79 mg (45 mg base)/wk x 8 wks	0.3 mg base/kg/d x 14d

64. Exchange transfusion has been helpful for some patients with high-density (>10%) parasitemia, altered mental status, pulmonary edema or renal complications (KD Miller et al, N Engl J Med 1989; 321:65).
65. Continuous EKG, blood pressure and glucose monitoring are recommended, especially in pregnant women and young children. For problems with quinidine availability, call the manufacturer (Eli Lilly, 800-821-0538) or the CDC Malaria Hotline (770-488-7788). Quinidine may have greater antimalarial activity than quinine. The loading dose should be decreased or omitted in those patients who have received quinine or mefloquine. If more than 48 hours of parenteral treatment is required, the quinine or quinidine dose should be reduced by 1/3 to 1/2.
66. Artemether-Quinine Meta-Analysis Study Group, Trans R Soc Trop Med Hyg 2001; 95:637. Not available in the US.
67. Relapses have been reported with this regimen, and should be treated with a second 14-day course of 30 mg base/day. In Southeast Asia and Somalia the higher dose (30 mg base/day) should be used initially.

Infection	Drug	Adult dosage	Pediatric dosage
MALARIA, Prevention of[68]			
Chloroquine-sensitive areas[49]			
Drug of choice:	Chloroquine phosphate[69,70]	500 mg (300 mg base), once/week[71]	5 mg/kg base once/week, up to adult dose of 300 mg base[71]
Chloroquine-resistant areas[49]			
Drug of choice:	Mefloquine[56,70,72]	250 mg once/week[71]	<15 kg: 5 mg/kg[71] 15-19 kg: ¼ tablet[71] 20-30 kg: ½ tablet[71] 31-45 kg: ¾ tablet[71] >45 kg: 1 tablet[71]
	OR Doxycycline[7, 70]	100 mg daily[73]	2 mg/kg/d, up to 100 mg/day[73]
	OR Atovaquone/ Proguanil[53,70]	250 mg/100 mg (1 adult tablet) daily[74]	11-20 kg: 62.5 mg/25 mg[74] 21-30 kg: 125 mg/50 mg[74] 31-40 kg: 187.5 mg/75 mg[74] >40 kg: 250 mg/100 mg[74]
Alternatives:	Primaquine[7,62,75]	30 mg base daily	0.5 mg/kg base daily

* Availability problems. See table on page 12.

68. No drug regimen guarantees protection against malaria. If fever develops within a year (particularly within the first two months) after travel to malarious areas, travelers should be advised to seek medical attention. Insect repellents, insecticide-impregnated bed nets and proper clothing are important adjuncts for malaria prophylaxis.
69. In pregnancy, chloroquine prophylaxis has been used extensively and safely.
70. For prevention of attack after departure from areas where *P. vivax* and *P. ovale* are endemic, which includes almost all areas where malaria is found (except Haiti), some experts prescribe in addition primaquine phosphate 26.3 mg (15 mg base)/d or, for children, 0.3 mg base/kg/d during the last two weeks of prophylaxis. Others prefer to avoid the toxicity of primaquine and rely on surveillance to detect cases when they occur, particularly when exposure was limited or doubtful. See also footnotes 62 and 67.
71. Beginning one to two weeks before travel and continuing weekly for the duration of stay and for four weeks after leaving.
72. The pediatric dosage has not been approved by the FDA, and the drug has not been approved for use during pregnancy. However, it has been reported to be safe for prophylactic use during the second or third trimester of pregnancy and possibly during early pregnancy as well (CDC Health Information for International Travel, 2001-2002, page 113; BL Smoak et al, J Infect Dis 1997; 176:831). Mefloquine is not recommended for patients with cardiac conduction abnormalities. Patients with a history of seizures or psychiatric disorders should avoid mefloquine (Medical Letter 1990; 32:13). Resistance to mefloquine has been reported in some areas, such as Thailand; in these areas, doxycycline should be used for prophylaxis. In children less than eight years old, proguanil plus sulfisoxazole has been used (KN Suh and JS Keystone, Infect Dis Clin Pract 1996; 5:541).

Infection	Drug	Adult dosage	Pediatric dosage
MALARIA, Prevention of *(continued)*			
Chloroquine-resistant areas[49]			
Alternatives:	Chloroquine phosphate	500 mg (300 mg base) once/week[71]	5 mg/kg base once/week, up to adult dose of 300 mg base[71]
	plus proguanil[76]	200 mg once/day	<2 yrs: 50 mg once/day 2-6 yrs: 100 mg once/day 7-10 yrs: 150 mg once/day >10 yrs: 200 mg once/day
Presumptive treatment	Atovaquone/ proguanil[53]	2 adult tablets bid x 3d[74]	11-20 kg: 1 adult tablet/day x 3 d[74] 21-30 kg: 2 adult tablets/day x 3 d[74] 31-40 kg: 3 adult tablets/day x 3 d[74] >40 kg: 2 adult tablets bid x 3 d[74]
	OR Pyrimethamine-sulfadoxine[51]	Carry a single dose (3 tablets) for self treatment of febrile illness when medical care is not immediately available	<1 yr: ¼ tablet 1-3 yrs: ½ tablet 4-8 yrs: 1 tablet 9-14 yrs: 2 tablets

73. Beginning 1-2 days before travel and continuing for the duration of stay and for 4 weeks after leaving. Use of tetracyclines is contraindicated in pregnancy and in children less than eight years old. Doxycycline can cause gastrointestinal disturbances, vaginal moniliasis and photosensitivity reactions.
74. GE Shanks et al, Clin Infect Dis 1998; 27:494; B Lell et al, Lancet 1998; 351:709. Beginning 1 to 2 days before travel and continuing for the duration of stay and for 1 week after leaving. In one study of malaria prophylaxis, atovaquone/proguanil was better tolerated than mefloquine in nonimmune travelers (D Overbosch et al, Clin Infect Dis 2001; 33:1015).
75. Several studies have shown that daily primaquine beginning one day before departure and continued until 7 days after leaving the malaria area provides effective prophylaxis against chloroquine-resistant *P. falciparum* (JK Baird et al, Clin Infect Dis 2001; 33:1990). Some studies have shown less efficacy against *P. vivax.* Nausea and abdominal pain can be diminished by taking with food.
76. Proguanil (*Paludrine* – Wyeth Ayerst, Canada; AstraZeneca, United Kingdom), which is not available alone in the US but is widely available in Canada and Europe, is recommended mainly for use in Africa south of the Sahara. Prophylaxis is recommended during exposure and for four weeks afterwards. Proguanil has been used in pregnancy without evidence of toxicity (PA Phillips-Howard and D Wood, Drug Saf 1996; 14:131).

Infection	Drug	Adult dosage	Pediatric dosage
MICROSPORIDIOSIS			
Ocular (*Encephalitozoon hellem, Encephalitozoon cuniculi, Vittaforma corneae* [*Nosema corneum*])			
Drug of choice:	Albendazole[7] plus fumagillin[77]*	400 mg bid	
Intestinal (*Enterocytozoon bieneusi, Encephalitozoon [Septata] intestinalis*)			
E. bieneusi[78]			
Drug of choice:	Fumagillin*	60 mg/d PO x 14d	
E. intestinalis			
Drug of choice:	Albendazole[7]	400 mg bid x 21d	
Disseminated (*E. hellem, E. cuniculi, E. intestinalis, Pleistophora sp., Trachipleistophora sp.* and *Brachiola vesicularum*)			
Drug of choice:[79]	Albendazole[7]	400 mg bid	
Mites, see SCABIES			
MONILIFORMIS *moniliformis* infection			
Drug of choice:	Pyrantel pamoate[7]	11 mg/kg once, repeat twice, 2 wks apart	11 mg/kg once, repeat twice, 2 wks apart
***Naegleria* species**, see AMEBIC MENINGOENCEPHALITIS, PRIMARY			
Necator americanus, see HOOKWORM infection			
OESOPHAGOSTOMUM *bifurcum*			
Drug of choice:	See footnote 80		
Onchocerca volvulus, see FILARIASIS			
Opisthorchis viverrini, see FLUKE infection			
Paragonimus westermani, see FLUKE infection			
Pediculus capitis, humanus, Phthirus pubis, see LICE			
Pinworm, see ENTEROBIUS			

* Availability problems. See table on page 12.

77. Ocular lesions due to *E. hellem* in HIV-infected patients have responded to fumagillin eyedrops prepared from *Fumidil-B*, a commercial product (Mid-Continent Agrimarketing, Inc., Olathe, Kansas, 800-547-1392) used to control a microsporidial disease of honey bees (MC Diesenhouse, Am J Ophthalmol 1993; 115:293). For lesions due to *V. corneae*, topical therapy is generally not effective and keratoplasty may be required (RM Davis et al, Ophthalmology 1990; 97:953).
78. Oral fumagillin (see footnote 76, Sanofi Recherche, Gentilly, France) has been effective in treating *E. bieneusi* (J-M Molina et al, AIDS 2000; 14:1341), but has been associated with thrombocytopenia. Highly active antiretroviral therapy (HAART) may lead to microbiologic and clinical response in HIV-infected patients with microsporidial diarrhea (NA Foudraine et al, AIDS 1998; 12:35; A Carr et al, Lancet 1998; 351:256). Octreotide *(Sandostatin)* has provided symptomatic relief in some patients with large volume diarrhea.
79. J-M Molina et al, J Infect Dis 1995; 171:245. There is no established treatment for *Pleistophora.*
80. Albendazole or pyrantel pamoate may be effective (HP Krepel et al, Trans R Soc Trop Med Hyg 1993; 87:87).

Infection	Drug	Adult dosage	Pediatric dosage
***PNEUMOCYSTIS** carinii* pneumonia (PCP)[81]			
Drug of choice:	Trimethoprim-sulfamethoxazole	TMP 15 mg/kg/d, SMX 75 mg/kg/d, oral or IV in 3 or 4 doses x 14-21d	Same as adult dose
Alternatives:	Primaquine[7,62]	30 mg base PO daily x 21 days	
	plus clindamycin[7]	600 mg IV q6h x 21 days, or 300-450 mg PO q6h x 21 days	
	OR Trimethoprim[7]	5 mg/kg PO tid x 21 days	
	plus dapsone[7]	100 mg PO daily x 21 days	
	Pentamidine	3-4 mg/kg IV daily x 14-21 days	Same as adult dose
	OR Atovaquone	750 mg bid PO x 21d	
Primary and secondary prophylaxis[82]			
Drug of Choice:	Trimethoprim-sulfamethoxazole	1 tab (single or double strength) daily	TMP 150 mg/m^2, SMX 750 mg/m^2 in 2 doses on 3 consecutive days per week
Alternatives:[83]	Dapsone[7]	50 mg bid, or 100 mg daily	2 mg/kg (max. 100 mg) daily or 4 mg/kg (max. 200 mg each week)
	OR Dapsone[7]	50 mg daily or 200 mg each week	
	plus pyrimethamine[84]	50 mg or 75 mg each week	

81. In severe disease with room air $PO_2 \leq 70$ mmHg or Aa gradient ≥ 35 mmHg, prednisone should also be used (S Gagnon et al, N Engl J Med 1990; 323:1444; E Caumes et al, Clin Infect Dis 1994; 18:319).
82. Primary/secondary prophylaxis in patients with HIV can be discontinued after CD4 count increases to >200 x 10^6/L for more than 3 months (HIV/AIDS Treatment Information Service, US Department of Health and Human Services 2001; www.hivatis.org).
83. An alternative trimethoprim/sulfamethoxazole regimen is one DS tab 3x/week. Weekly therapy with sulfadoxine 500 mg/pyrimethamine 25 mg/leucovorin 25 mg was effective PCP prophylaxis in liver transplant patients (J Torre-Cisneros et al, Clin Infect Dis 1999; 29:771).
84. Plus leucovorin 25 mg with each dose of pyrimethamine.

Infection	Drug	Adult dosage	Pediatric dosage
Primary and secondary prophylaxis[82] *(continued)*			
	OR Pentamidine aerosol	300 mg inhaled monthly via *Respirgard II* nebulizer	≥5 yrs: same as adult dose
	OR Atovaquone[7]	1500 mg daily	
Roundworm, see ASCARIASIS			
Sappinia Diploidea, See AMEBIC MENINGOENCEPHALITIS, PRIMARY			
SCABIES *(Sarcoptes scabiei)*			
Drug of choice:	5% Permethrin	Topically	Topically
Alternatives:	Ivermectin[7,85]	200 µg/kg PO once	200 µg/kg PO once
	10% Crotamiton	Topically once/daily x 2	Topically once/daily x 2
SCHISTOSOMIASIS *(Bilharziasis)*			
S. haematobium			
Drug of choice:	Praziquantel	40 mg/kg/d in 2 doses x 1d	40 mg/kg/d in 2 doses x 1d
S. japonicum			
Drug of choice:	Praziquantel	60 mg/kg/d in 3 doses x 1d	60 mg/kg/d in 3 doses x 1d
S. mansoni			
Drug of choice:	Praziquantel	40 mg/kg/d in 2 doses x 1d	40 mg/kg/d in 2 doses x 1d
Alternative:	Oxamniquine[86]	15 mg/kg once[87]	20 mg/kg/d in 2 doses x 1d[87]
S. mekongi			
Drug of choice:	Praziquantel	60 mg/kg/d in 3 doses x 1d	60 mg/kg/d in 3 doses x 1d
Sleeping sickness, see TRYPANOSOMIASIS			
STRONGYLOIDIASIS *(Strongyloides stercoralis)*			
Drug of choice:[88]	Ivermectin	200 µg/kg/d x 1-2d	200 µg/kg/d x 1-2d
Alternative:	Thiabendazole	50 mg/kg/d in 2 doses (max. 3 grams/d) x 2d[89]	50 mg/kg/d in 2 doses (max. 3 grams/d) x 2d[89]

* Availability problems. See table on page 12.

85. Effective for crusted scabies in immunocompromised patients (M Larralde et al, Pediatr Dermatol 1999; 16:69; A Patel et al, Australas J Dermatol 1999; 40:37; O Chosidow, Lancet 2000; 355:819).
86. Oxamniquine has been effective in some areas in which praziquantel is less effective (FF Stelma et al, J Infect Dis 1997; 176:304). Oxamniquine is contraindicated in pregnancy.
87. In East Africa, the dose should be increased to 30 mg/kg, and in Egypt and South Africa to 30 mg/kg/d x 2d. Some experts recommend 40-60 mg/kg over 2-3 days in all of Africa (KC Shekhar, Drugs 1991; 42:379).

Infection	Drug	Adult dosage	Pediatric dosage
TAPEWORM infection			
— Adult (intestinal stage)			
***Diphyllobothrium latum* (fish), *Taenia saginata* (beef), *Taenia solium* (pork), *Dipylidium caninum* (dog)**			
Drug of choice:	Praziquantel[7]	5-10 mg/kg once	5-10 mg/kg once
Alternative:	Niclosamide	2 g once	50 mg/kg once
***Hymenolepis nana* (dwarf tapeworm)**			
Drug of choice:	Praziquantel[7]	25 mg/kg once	25 mg/kg once
— Larval (tissue stage)			
***Echinococcus granulosus* (hydatid cyst)**			
Drug of choice:[90]	Albendazole	400 mg bid x 1-6 months	15 mg/kg/d (max. 800 mg) x 1-6 months
Echinococcus multilocularis			
Treatment of choice:	See footnote 91		
***Cysticercus cellulosae* (cysticercosis)**			
Treatment of choice:	See footnote 92		
Alternative:	Albendazole	400 mg bid x 8-30d; can be repeated as necessary	15 mg/kg/d (max. 800 mg) in 2 doses x 8-30d; can be repeated as necessary
	OR Praziquantel[7]	50-100 mg/kg/d in 3 doses x 30d	50-100 mg/kg/d in 3 doses x 30d

88. In immunocompromised patients or disseminated disease, it may be necessary to prolong or repeat therapy or use other agents. A veterinary parenteral formulation of ivermectin was used in one patient (PL Chiodini et al, Lancet 2000; 355:43).
89. This dose is likely to be toxic and may have to be decreased.
90. Patients may benefit from or require surgical resection of cysts. Praziquantel is useful preoperatively or in case of spill during surgery. Percutaneous drainage with ultrasound guidance plus albendazole therapy has been effective for management of hepatic hydatid cyst disease (MS Khuroo et al, N Engl J Med 1997; 337:881; O Akhan and M Ozman, Eur J Radiol 1999; 32:76).
91. Surgical excision or the PAIR (Puncture, Aspirate, Inject, Re-aspirate) technique is the only reliable means of cure. Reports have suggested that in non-resectable cases use of albendazole or mebendazole can stabilize and sometimes cure infection (W Hao et al, Trans R Soc Trop Med Hyg 1994; 88:340; WHO Group, Bull WHO 1996; 74:231).
92. Initial therapy of parenchymal disease with seizures should focus on symptomatic treatment with anticonvulsant drugs. Treatment of parenchymal disease with albendazole and praziquantel is controversial and randomized trials have not been conclusive. Obstructive hydrocephalus is treated with surgical removal of the obstructing cyst or CSF diversion. Prednisone 40 mg daily may be given in conjunction with surgery. Arachnoiditis, vasculitis or cerebral edema is treated with prednisone 60 mg daily or dexamethasone 4-16 mg/d combined with albendazole or praziquantel (AC White, Jr, Annu Rev Med 2000; 51:187). Patients with subarachnoid cysts or giant cysts in the fissures should receive albendazole for at least 30 days (JV Proano et al, N Engl J Med 2001; 345:879). Any cysticercocidal drug may cause irreparable damage when used to treat ocular or spinal cysts, even when corticosteroids are used. An ophthalmic exam should always be done before treatment to rule out intraocular cysts.

Infection	Drug	Adult dosage	Pediatric dosage
Toxocariasis, see VISCERAL LARVA MIGRANS			
TOXOPLASMOSIS *(Toxoplasma gondii)*[93]			
Drugs of choice:[94]	Pyrimethamine[95]	25-100 mg/d x 3-4 wks	2 mg/kg/d x 3d, (max. 25 mg/d) x 4 wks[96]
	plus sulfadiazine	1-1.5 grams qid x 3-4 wks	100-200 mg/kg/d x 3-4 wks
Alternative:[97]	Spiramycin*	3-4 grams/d x 3-4 wks	50-100 mg/kg/d x 3-4 wks
TRICHINOSIS *(Trichinella spiralis)*			
Drugs of choice:	Steroids for severe symptoms		
	plus mebendazole[7]	200-400 mg tid x 3d, then 400-500 mg tid x 10d	200-400 mg tid x 3d, then 400-500 mg tid x 10d
Alternative:	Albendazole[7]	400 mg bid x 8-14d	400 mg bid x 8-14d

* Availability problems. See table on page 12.

93. In ocular toxoplasmosis with macular involvement, corticosteroids are recommended for an anti-inflammatory effect on the eyes.
94. To treat CNS toxoplasmosis in HIV-infected patients, some clinicians have used pyrimethamine 50 to 100 mg daily (after a loading dose of 200 mg) with sulfadiazine and, when sulfonamide sensitivity developed, have given clindamycin 1.8 to 2.4 g/d in divided doses instead of the sulfonamide (JS Remington et al, Lancet 1991; 338:1142; BJ Luft et al, N Engl J Med 1993; 329:995). Atovaquone plus pyrimethamine appears to be an effective alternative in sulfa-intolerant patients (JA Kovacs et al, Lancet 1992; 340:637). Treatment is followed by chronic suppression with lower dosage regimens of the same drugs. For primary prophylaxis in HIV patients with <100 CD4 cells, either trimethoprim-sulfamethoxazole, pyrimethamine with dapsone or atovaquone with or without pyrimethamine can be used. Primary/Secondary prophylaxis may be discontinued when the CD4 count increases to >200 x 10^6/L for more than 3 months (HIV/AIDS Treatment Information Service US Department of Health and Human Services 2001; (www.hivatis.org). See also footnote 95.
95. Plus leucovorin 10 to 25 mg with each dose of pyrimethamine.
96. Congenitally infected newborns should be treated with pyrimethamine every two or three days and a sulfonamide daily for about one year (JS Remington and G Desmonts in JS Remington and JO Klein, eds, *Infectious Disease of the Fetus and Newborn Infant*, 5th ed, Philadelphia:Saunders, 2001, page 290).
97. For prophylactic use during pregnancy. If it is determined that transmission has occurred *in utero*, therapy with pyrimethamine and sulfadiazine should be started. Pyrimethamine is a potential teratogen and should be used only after the first trimester.
98. Sexual partners should be treated simultaneously. Metronidazole-resistant strains have been reported and should be treated with metronidazole 2-4 g/d x 7-14d. Desensitization has been recommended for patients allergic to metronidazole (MD Pearlman et al, Am J Obstet Gynecol 1996; 174:934). High dose tinidazole has also been used for the treatment of metronidazole-resistant trichomoniasis (JD Sobel et al, Clin Infect Dis 2001; 33:1341).

Infection	Drug	Adult dosage	Pediatric dosage
TRICHOMONIASIS *(Trichomonas vaginalis)*			
Drug of choice:[98]	Metronidazole	2 grams once or 500 mg bid x 7d	15 mg/kg/d orally in 3 doses x 7d
	OR Tinidazole[5]	2 grams once or 500 mg bid	50 mg/kg once (max. 2 g)
TRICHOSTRONGYLUS infection			
Drug of choice:	Pyrantel pamoate[7]	11 mg/kg base once (max. 1 g)	11 mg/kg once (max. 1 gram)
Alternative:	Mebendazole[7]	100 mg bid x 3d	100 mg bid x 3d
	OR Albendazole[7]	400 mg once	400 mg once
TRICHURIASIS (*Trichuris trichiura*, whipworm)			
Drug of choice:	Mebendazole	100 mg bid x 3d or 500 mg once	100 mg bid x 3d or 500 mg once
Alternative:	Albendazole[7]	400 mg x 3d	400 mg x 3d
TRYPANOSOMIASIS			
T. cruzi **(American trypanosomiasis, Chagas' disease)**			
Drug of choice:	Benznidazole*	5-7 mg/kg/d in 2 divided doses x 30-90d	Up to 12 yrs: 10 mg/kg/d in 2 doses x 30-90d
	OR Nifurtimox[99]*	8-10 mg/kg/d in 3-4 doses x 90-120d	1-10 yrs: 15-20 mg/kg/d in 4 doses x 90d; 11-16 yrs: 12.5-15 mg/kg/d in 4 doses x 90d
T. brucei gambiense **(West African trypanosomiasis, sleeping sickness) hemolymphatic stage**			
Drug of choice:[100]	Pentamidine isethionate[7]	4 mg/kg/d IM x 10d	4 mg/kg/d IM x 10d
Alternative:	Suramin*	100-200 mg (test dose) IV, then 1 gram IV on days 1,3,7,14, and 21	20 mg/kg on days 1,3,7,14, and 21
	OR Eflornithine*	See footnote 101	

99. Available from CDC. The addition of gamma interferon to nifurtimox for 20 days in a limited number of patients and in experimental animals appears to have shortened the acute phase of Chagas' disease (RE McCabe et al, J Infect Dis 1991; 163:912).

100. For treatment of *T.b. gambiense*, pentamidine and suramin have equal efficacy but pentamidine is better tolerated.

101. Eflornithine is highly effective in *T.b. gambiense* and variably effective in *T. b. rhodesiense* infections. It is available in limited supply only from the WHO, and is given 400 mg/kg/d IV in 4 divided doses for 14 days.

Infection	Drug	Adult dosage	Pediatric dosage
T. b. rhodesiense **(East African trypanosomiasis, sleeping sickness) hemolymphatic stage**			
Drug of choice:	Suramin*	100-200 mg (test dose) IV, then 1 gram IV on days 1,3,7,14, and 21	20 mg/kg on days 1,3,7,14, and 21
late disease with CNS involvement *(T.b. gambiense or T.b. rhodesiense)*			
Drug of choice:	Melarsoprol[102]*	2-3.6 mg/kg/d IV x 3d; after 1 wk 3.6 mg/kg per day IV x 3d; repeat again after 10-21 days	18-25 mg/kg total over 1 month; initial dose of 0.36 mg/kg IV, increasing gradually to max. 3.6 mg/kg at intervals of 1-5d for total of 9-10 doses
OR	Eflornithine	See footnote 101	
VISCERAL LARVA MIGRANS[103] (Toxocariasis)			
Drug of choice:	Albendazole[7]	400 mg bid x 5d	400 mg bid x 5d
	Mebendazole[7]	100-200 mg bid x 5d	100-200 mg bid x 5d
Whipworm, see TRICHURIASIS			
Wuchereria bancrofti, see FILARIASIS			

* Availability problems. See table on page 12.

102. In frail patients, begin with as little as 18 mg and increase the dose progressively. Pretreatment with suramin has been advocated for debilitated patients. Corticosteroids have been used to prevent arsenical encephalopathy (J Pepin et al, Trans R Soc Trop Med Hyg 1995; 89:92). Up to 20% of patients with *T. gambiense* fail to respond to melarsoprol (MP Barrett, Lancet 1999; 353:1113). A shortened course consisting of 10 daily injections of 2.2 mg/kg gave a similar outcome to the usual 26-treatment schedule (C Burri et al, Lancet 2000; 355:1419).

103. Optimum duration of therapy is not known; some Medical Letter consultants would treat for up to 20 days. For severe symptoms or eye involvement, corticosteroids can be used in addition.

MANUFACTURERS OF SOME ANTIPARASITIC DRUGS

albendazole – *Albenza* (GlaxoSmithKline)
§ artemether – *Artenam* (Arenco, Belgium)
§ artesunate – (Guilin No. 1 Factory, People's Republic of China)
atovaquone – *Mepron* (GlaxoSmithKline)
atovaquone/proguanil — *Malarone* (GlaxoSmithKline)
bacitracin – many manufacturers
§ bacitracin-zinc – (Apothekernes Laboratorium A.S., Oslo, Norway)
§ benznidazole – *Rochagan* (Roche, Brazil)
† bithionol – *Bitin* (Tanabe, Japan)
chloroquine HCl and chloroquine phosphate – *Aralen* (Sanofi), others
crotamiton – *Eurax* (Westwood-Squibb)
dapsone – (Jacobus)
† diethylcarbamazine citrate USP – (University of Iowa School of Pharmacy)
§ diloxanide furoate – *Furamide* (Boots, United Kingdom)
§ eflornithine (Difluoromethylornithine, DFMO) – *Ornidyl* (Aventis)
furazolidone – *Furoxone* (Roberts)
§ halofantrine – *Halfan* (GlaxoSmithKline)
iodoquinol – *Yodoxin* (Glenwood), others
ivermectin – *Stromectol* (Merck)
malathion – *Ovide* (Medicis)
mebendazole – *Vermox* (McNeil)
mefloquine – *Lariam* (Roche)
§ meglumine antimonate – *Glucantime* (Aventis, France)
† melarsoprol – *Mel-B* (Specia)
metronidazole – *Flagyl* (Searle), others
§ miltefosine – (Zentaris)
§ niclosamide – *Yomesan* (Bayer, Germany)
† nifurtimox – *Lampit* (Bayer, Germany)
* nitazoxanide – *Cryptaz* (Romark)
§ ornidazole – *Tiberal* (Roche, France)
oxamniquine – *Vansil* (Pfizer)
paromomycin – *Humatin* (Monarch); *Leshcutan* (Teva Pharmaceutical Industries, Ltd., Israel; topical formulation not available in US)
pentamidine isethionate – *Pentam 300, NebuPent* (Fujisawa)
permethrin – *Nix* (GlaxoSmithKline), *Elimite* (Allergan)
praziquantel – *Biltricide* (Bayer)
primaquine phosphate USP
§ proguanil – *Paludrine* (Wyeth Ayerst, Canada; AstraZeneca, United Kingdom); in combination with atovaquone as *Malarone* (GlaxoSmithKline)
§ propamidine isethionate – *Brolene* (Aventis, Canada)
pyrantel pamoate – *Antiminth* (Pfizer)
pyrethrins and piperonyl butoxide – *RID* (Pfizer), others
pyrimethamine USP – *Daraprim* (GlaxoSmithKline)
§ quinine dihydrochloride
quinine sulfate – many manufacturers
† sodium stibogluconate – *Pentostam* (GlaxoSmithKline, United Kingdom)
* spiramycin – *Rovamycine* (Aventis)
† suramin sodium – (Bayer, Germany)
thiabendazole – *Mintezol* (Merck)
§ tinidazole – *Fasigyn* (Pfizer)
* triclabendazole – *Egaten* (Novartis, Switzerland)
trimetrexate – *Neutrexin* (US Bioscience)

---

* Available in the US only from the manufacturer.
§ Not available in the US.
† Available under an Investigational New Drug (IND) protocol from the CDC Drug Service, Centers for Disease Control and Prevention, Atlanta, Georgia 30333; 404-639-3670 (evenings, weekends, or holidays: 404-639-2888).

PRINCIPAL ADVERSE EFFECTS OF ANTIMICROBIAL DRUGS

Adverse effects of antimicrobial drugs vary with dosage, duration of administration, concomitant therapy, renal and hepatic function, immune competence, and the age of the patient. The principal adverse effects of antimicrobial agents are listed in the following table. The designation of adverse effects as "frequent," "occasional" or "rare" is based on published reports and on the experience of Medical Letter consultants. Information about adverse interactions between drugs, including probable mechanisms and recommendations for clinical management, are available in the current edition of *The Medical Letter Handbook of Adverse Drug Interactions* and in the Medical Letter *Adverse Drug Interactions Program*.

ABACAVIR *(Ziagen)*
Frequent: hypersensitivity reaction with fever, GI or respiratory symptoms and rash
Occasional: arthralgias; anemia; lactic acidosis
Rare: anaphylaxis; pancreatitis; hyperglycemia

ACYCLOVIR *(Zovirax*; others)
Frequent: local irritation at infusion site
Occasional: local reactions with topical use; headache, rash, nausea, diarrhea, vertigo, and arthralgias with oral use; decreased renal function sometimes progressing to renal failure; metabolic encephalopathy; bone marrow depression; abnormal hepatic function in immunocompromised patients
Rare: lethargy or agitation; tremor; disorientation; hallucinations; transient hemiparesthesia

ALBENDAZOLE *(Albenza)*
Occasional: abdominal pain; reversible alopecia; increased serum transaminase activity; migration of ascaris through mouth and nose
Rare: leukopenia; rash; renal toxicity

AMANTADINE (*Symmetrel*, others)
Frequent: livedo reticularis and ankle edema; insomnia; dizziness; lethargy
Occasional: depression; psychosis; confusion; slurred speech; congestive heart failure; orthostatic hypotension; urinary retention; GI disturbance; rash; visual disturbance; sudden loss of vision; increased seizures in epilepsy
Rare: convulsions; leukopenia; neutropenia; eczematoid dermatitis; oculogyric episodes; photosensitivity

AMIKACIN *(Amikin)*
Occasional: vestibular damage; renal damage; fever; rash
Rare: auditory damage; CNS reactions; blurred vision; nausea; vomiting; neuromuscular blockade and apnea, may be reversible with calcium salts; paresthesias; hypotension

AMINOSALICYLIC ACID *(Paser)*
Frequent: GI disturbance
Occasional: allergic reactions; liver damage; renal irritation; blood dyscrasias; thyroid enlargement; malabsorption syndrome
Rare: acidosis; hypokalemia; encephalopathy; vasculitis; hypoglycemia in diabetics

AMOXICILLIN — See Penicillins

AMOXICILLIN/CLAVULANIC ACID — See Penicillins

AMPHOTERICIN B DEOXYCHOLATE (*Fungizone*, others)
Frequent: renal damage; hypokalemia; thrombophlebitis at site of peripheral vein infusion; anorexia; headache; nausea; weight loss; bone marrow suppression with reversible decline in hematocrit; chills, fever, vomiting during infusion, possibly with delirium, hypotension or hypertension, wheezing, and hypoxemia, especially in cardiac or pulmonary disease
Occasional: hypomagnesemia; normocytic, normochromic anemia
Rare: hemorrhagic gastroenteritis; blood dyscrasias; rash; blurred vision; peripheral neuropathy; convulsions; anaphylaxis; arrhythmias; acute liver failure; reversible nephrogenic diabetes insipidus; hearing loss; acute pulmonary edema; spinal cord damage with intrathecal use

AMPHOTERICIN B LIPID FORMULATIONS *(Ambisone, Abelcet, Amphotec)* — See page 114.

AMPICILLIN — See Penicillins

AMPICILLIN/SULBACTAM — See Penicillins

AMPRENAVIR *(Agenerase)*
Frequent: GI disturbance; oral and perioral paresthesias; rash; hypersensitivity with fever
Occasional: hyperglycemia; increased aminotransferase activity; hyperlipidemia; abnormal fat distribution
Rare: severe rash including Stevens-Johnson syndrome; hemolytic anemia

ARTEMETHER *(Artenam)*
Occasional: neurological toxicity; possible increase in length of coma; increased convulsions; prolongation of QTc interval

ARTESUNATE
Occasional: ataxia; slurred speech; neurological toxicity; possible increase in length of coma; increased convulsions; prolongation of QTc interval

ATOVAQUONE *(Mepron, Malarone* [with proguanil])
Frequent: rash; nausea
Occasional: diarrhea; increased aminotransferase activity; cholestasis

AZITHROMYCIN *(Zithromax)*
Occasional: nausea; diarrhea; abdominal pain; headache; dizziness; vaginitis
Rare: angioedema; cholestatic jaundice; photosensitivity; reversible dose-related hearing loss

AZT — See Zidovudine

AZTREONAM *(Azactam)*
Occasional: local reaction at injection site; rash; diarrhea; nausea; vomiting; increased aminotransferase activity
Rare: thrombocytopenia; pseudomembranous colitis

BACITRACIN — many manufacturers
Frequent: nephrotoxicity; GI disturbance
Occasional: rash; blood dyscrasias
Rare: anaphylaxis

BENZNIDAZOLE *(Rochagan)*
Frequent: allergic rash; dose-dependent polyneuropathy; GI disturbance; psychic disturbances

BITHIONOL *(Bitin)*
Frequent: photosensitivity reactions; votmiting; diarrhea; abdominal pain; urticaria
Rare: leukopenia; toxic hepatitis

CAPREOMYCIN *(Capastat)*
Occasional: renal damage; eighth-nerve damage; hypokalemia and other electrolyte abnormalities; pain, induration, excessive bleeding, sterile abscess at injection site
Rare: allergic reactions; leukocytosis, leukopenia; neuromuscular blockade and apnea with large IV doses, reversed by neostigmine

CARBENICILLIN — See Penicillins

CASPOFUNGIN *(Cancidas)*
Occasional: fever; rash; increased aminotransferase activity; GI disturbance; facial flushing
Rare: anaphylaxis

CEPHALOSPORINS
(cefaclor – *Ceclor*; cefadroxil – *Duricef*, others; cefamandole – *Mandol*; cefazolin – *Ancef*, others; cefdinir – *Omnicef*; cefditoren pivoxil – *Spectracef*; cefepime – *Maxipime*; cefixime – *Suprax*; cefonicid – *Monocid*; cefoperazone – *Cefobid*; cefotaxime – *Claforan*; cefotetan – *Cefotan*; cefoxitin – *Mefoxin*; cefpodoxime – *Vantin*; cefprozil – *Cefzil*; ceftazidime – *Fortaz, Tazidime, Tazicef, Ceptaz*; ceftibuten – *Cedax*; ceftizoxime – *Cefizox*; ceftriaxone – *Rocephin*; cefuroxime – *Kefurox, Zinacef*; cefuroxime axetil – *Ceftin*; cephalexin – *Keflex*, others; cephapirin – *Cefadyl*, others; cephradine – *Velosef*, others; loracarbef – *Lorabid*
Frequent: thrombophlebitis with IV use; serum-sickness-like reaction with prolonged parenteral administration; moderate to severe diarrhea, especially with cefoperazone and cefixime
Occasional: allergic reactions, rarely anaphylactic; pain at injection site; GI disturbance; hypoprothrombinemia, hemorrhage with cefamandole, cefoperazone or cefotetan; rash and arthritis ("serum-sickness") with cefaclor or cefprozil, especially in children; cholelithiasis with ceftriaxone; vaginal candidiasis (especially with cefdinir); carnitine deficiency with prolonged use of cefditoren
Rare: hemolytic anemia; hepatic dysfunction; blood dyscrasias; renal damage; acute interstitial nephritis; pseudomembranous colitis; seizures; toxic epidermal necrolysis

CHLORAMPHENICOL
(*Chloromycetin*, others)
Occasional: blood dyscrasias; gray syndrome (cardiovascular collapse); GI disturbance
Rare: fatal aplastic anemia, even with eye drops or ointment; allergic and febrile reactions; peripheral neuropathy; optic neuritis and other CNS injury; pseudomembranous colitis

CHLOROQUINE HCL and CHLOROQUINE PHOSPHATE (*Aralen*, and others)
Occasional: pruritus; vomiting; headache; confusion; depigmentation of hair; skin eruptions; corneal opacity; weight loss; partial alopecia; extraocular muscle palsies; exacerbation of psoriasis, eczema, and other exfoliative dermatoses; myalgias; photophobia
Rare: irreversible retinal injury (especially when total dosage exceeds 100 grams); discoloration of nails and mucus membranes; nerve-type deafness; peripheral neuropathy and myopathy; heart block; blood dyscrasias; hematemesis

CIDOFOVIR *(Vistide)*
Frequent: nephrotoxicity; ocular hypotony; neutropenia
Occasional: metabolic acidosis; uveitis; Fanconi syndrome

CINOXACIN (*Cinobac*, others) — Probably same as nalidixic acid

CIPROFLOXACIN *(Cipro)* — See Fluoroquinolones

CLARITHROMYCIN *(Biaxin)*
Occasional: nausea; diarrhea; abdominal pain; abnormal taste; headache; dizziness
Rare: reversible dose-related hearing loss; pseudomembranous colitis; pancreatitis; torsades de pointes

CLINDAMYCIN (*Cleocin*, others)
Frequent: diarrhea; allergic reactions
Occasional: pseudomembranous colitis, sometimes severe, can occur even with topical use
Rare: blood dyscrasias; esophageal ulceration; hepatotoxicity; arrhythmia due to QTc prolongation

CLOFAZIMINE *(Lamprene)*
Frequent: ichthyosis; pigmentation of skin, cornea and retina; urine discoloration; dryness and irritation of eyes; GI disturbance
Occasional: headache; retinal degeneration
Rare: splenic infarction, bowel obstruction, and GI bleeding with high doses

CLOXACILLIN — See Penicillins

COLISTIMETHATE — See Polymyxins

CROTAMITON *(Eurax)*
Occasional: rash

CYCLOSERINE (*Seromycin*, others)
Frequent: anxiety; depression; confusion; disorientation; paranoia; hallucinations; somnolence; headache
Occasional: peripheral neuropathy; liver damage; malabsorption syndrome; folate deficiency
Rare: suicide; seizures; coma

DAPSONE
Frequent: rash; transient headache; GI irritation; anorexia; infectious mononucleosis-like syndrome
Occasional: cyanosis due to methemoglobinemia and sulfhemoglobinemia; other blood dyscrasias, including hemolytic anemia; nephrotic syndrome; liver damage; peripheral neuropathy; hypersensitivity reactions; increased risk of lepra reactions; insomnia; irritability; uncoordinated speech; agitation; acute psychosis
Rare: renal papillary necrosis; severe hypoalbuminemia; epidermal necrolysis; optic atrophy; agranulocytosis; neonatal hyperbilirubinemia after use in pregnancy

DELAVIRDINE *(Rescriptor)* — Similar to nevirapine, but rash may be less severe and hepatotoxicity is less common

DEMECLOCYCLINE — See Tetracyclines

DICLOXACILLIN — See Penicillins

DIDANOSINE (ddI; *Videx)*
Frequent: peripheral neuropathy; diarrhea; nausea; vomiting; abdominal pain
Occasional: pancreatitis; hyperuricemia; increased aminotransferase activity; hypokalemia; headache; constipation; loss of taste; fever; rash; lactic acidosis; retinal depigmentation
Rare: hepatic failure; retinal atrophy in children

DIETHYLCARBAMAZINE CITRATE *(Hetrazan)*
Frequent: severe allergic or febrile reactions in patients with microfilaria in the blood or the skin; GI disturbance
Rare: encephalopathy

DILOXANIDE FUROATE *(Furamide)*
Frequent: flatulence
Occasional: nausea; vomiting; diarrhea
Rare: diplopia; dizziness; urticaria; pruritus

DIRITHROMYCIN *(Dynabac)* — Similar to erythromycin

DOXYCYCLINE — See Tetracyclines

EFAVIRENZ *(Sustiva)*
Frequent: dizziness; headache; inability to concentrate; insomnia and somnolence; rash
Occasional: vivid dreams; nightmares; hallucinations; hypersensitivity reaction with fever, GI or respiratory symptoms and rash; Stevens-Johnson syndrome in children
Rare: pancreatitis; peripheral neuropathy; psychiatric symptoms; photosensitivity reactions

EFLORNITHINE (Difluoromethylornithine, DFMO, *Ornidyl*)
Frequent: anemia; leukopenia
Occasional: diarrhea; thrombocytopenia; seizures
Rare: hearing loss

ENOXACIN — See Fluoroquinolones

ERTAPENEM *(Invanz)*
Occasional: phlebitis; nausea; vomiting; diarrhea
Rare: seizures

ERYTHROMYCIN (*Ery-Tab*, others)
Frequent: GI disturbance
Occasional: stomatitis; cholestatic hepatitis especially with erythromycin estolate in adults
Rare: allergic reactions, including severe respiratory distress; pseudomembranous colitis; hemolytic anemia; hepatotoxicity; transient hearing loss with high doses, prolonged use, or in patients with renal insufficiency; ventricular arrhythmias including torsades de pointes with IV infusion; aggravation of myasthenia gravis; hypothermia; pancreatitis; hypertrophic pyloric stenosis following treatment of infants

ETHAMBUTOL *(Myambutol)*
Occasional: optic neuritis; allergic reactions; GI disturbance; mental confusion; precipitation of acute gout
Rare: peripheral neuritis; possible renal damage; thrombocytopenia; toxic epidermal necrolysis; lichenoid skin eruption

ETHIONAMIDE *(Trecator-SC)*
Frequent: GI disturbance
Occasional: liver damage; CNS disturbance, including peripheral neuropathy; allergic reactions; gynecomastia; depression; myalgias; hypotension
Rare: hypothyroidism; optic neuritis; arthritis; impotence

FAMCICLOVIR *(Famvir)*
Occasional: headache; nausea; diarrhea

FLUCONAZOLE *(Diflucan)*
Occasional: nausea; vomiting; diarrhea; abdominal pain; headache; rash; increased aminotransferase activity
Rare: severe hepatic toxicity; exfoliative dermatitis; anaphylaxis; Stevens-Johnson syndrome; toxic epidermal necrolysis; hair loss

FLUCYTOSINE *(Ancobon)*
Frequent: blood dyscrasias, including pancytopenia and fatal agranulocytosis; GI disturbance, including severe diarrhea and ulcerative colitis; rash; hepatic dysfunction
Occasional: confusion; hallucinations
Rare: anaphylaxis

FLUOROQUINOLONES
(ciprofloxacin – *Cipro*; enoxacin – *Penetrex*; gatifloxacin – *Tequin*; levofloxacin – *Levaquin*; lomefloxacin – *Maxaquin*; moxifloxacin – *Avelox*; norfloxacin – *Noroxin*; ofloxacin – *Floxin*)
Occasional: nausea; vomiting; abdominal pain; dizziness; headache; tremors; restlessness; confusion; rash; *Candida* infections of the pharynx and vagina; eosinophilia; neutropenia; increased hepatic enzyme activity; increased serum creatinine concentration; insomnia; diarrhea; leukopenia; photosensitivity reactions, especially with lomefloxacin; prolongation of QTc interval
Rare: hallucinations; delirium; psychosis; vertigo; paresthesias; blurred vision and photophobia; severe hepatitis; seizures; pseudomembranous colitis; interstitial nephritis; vasculitis; possible exacerbation of myasthenia gravis; serum-sickness-like reaction; anaphylaxis; toxic epidermal necrolysis; anemia; tendinitis or tendon rupture; ventricular tachycardia and torsades de pointes; rhabdomyolysis with ofloxacin

FOSCARNET *(Foscavir)*
Frequent: renal dysfunction; anemia; nausea; disturbances of Ca, P, Mg, and K metabolism
Occasional: headache; vomiting; fatigue; genital ulceration; seizures; neuropathy
Rare: Nephrogenic diabetes insipidus; cardiac arrhythmias; hypertension

FOSFOMYCIN *(Monurol)*
Frequent: diarrhea
Occasional: vaginitis

FURAZOLIDONE *(Furoxone)*
Frequent: nausea; vomiting
Occasional: allergic reactions, including pulmonary infiltration; hypotension; urticaria; fever; vesicular rash; hypoglycemia; headache
Rare: hemolytic anemia in G-6-PD deficiency and neonates; disulfiram-like reaction with alcohol; MAO-inhibitor interactions; polyneuritis

GANCICLOVIR *(Cytovene)*
Frequent: neutropenia; thrombocytopenia
Occasional: anemia; fever; rash; abnormal liver function; neurological toxicity; phlebitis
Rare: hypertension; cardiac arrhythmias; nausea; vomiting; abdominal pain; diarrhea; eosinophilia; hypoglycemia; alopecia; pruritus; urticaria; renal toxicity; psychiatric disturbances; seizures

GATIFLOXACIN — See Fluoroquinolones

GENTAMICIN (*Garamycin*, others)
Occasional: vestibular damage; renal damage; rash
Rare: auditory damage; neuromuscular blockade and apnea, reversible with calcium or neostigmine; disturbed mental function; polyneuropathy; anaphylaxis

GRISEOFULVIN (*Fulvicin-U/F*, others)
Occasional: GI disturbance; allergic and photosensitivity reactions
Rare: proteinuria; blood dyscrasias; mental confusion; paresthesias; exacerbation of lupus; fixed-drug eruption; reversible liver damage; lymphadenopathy; exacerbation of leprosy

HALOFANTRINE *(Halfan)*
Occasional: diarrhea; abdominal pain; pruritus; prolongation of QTc and PR interval
Rare: fatal cardiac arrhythmias

IMIPENEM-CILASTATIN *(Primaxin)*
Occasional: phlebitis; pain at injection site; fever; urticaria; rash; pruritus; nausea, vomiting and transient hypotension during intravenous infusion; diarrhea
Rare: seizures; pseudomembranous colitis

IMIQUIMOD *(Aldara)*
Frequent: local erythema, erosion and excoriation
Occasional: itching, burning and pain

INDINAVIR *(Crixivan)*
Frequent: hyperbilirubinemia; dysuria; kidney stones; flank pain; hematuria; crystalluria
Occasional: hemolytic anemia; increased aminotransferase activity; GI disturbance; reflux esophagitis; glucose intolerance; hyperlipidemia; abnormal fat distribution; increased bleeding in hemophiliacs; paronychia; alopecia; dry skin and mucous membranes
Rare: rash; hyperprolactinemia

INTERFERON ALFA *(Alferon N, Infergen, Intron A, Roferon-A, Rebetron* with ribavirin; Pegylated interferon alfa 2b – *Peg-Intron)*
Frequent: Transient flu-like syndrome; fatigue; anorexia; nausea; diarrhea; rash; dry skin or pruritus; weight loss; change in taste; bone marrow suppression; increased aminotransferase activity; depression; anxiety; insomnia
Occasional: Paresthesias; alopecia; diaphoresis; reactivation of herpes labialis; hypo- and hyperthyroidism; tinnitus; activation of auto-immune diseases, including diabetes
Rare: Visual disturbance and retinopathy; hypertension; cardiac arrhythmias; renal failure; nephrotic syndrome; hearing loss

IODOQUINOL (*Yodoxin*, others)
Occasional: rash; acne; slight enlargement of the thyroid gland; nausea; diarrhea; cramps; anal pruritus
Rare: optic neuritis, atrophy and loss of vision; peripheral neuropathy after prolonged use in high dosage (for months); iodine sensitivity

ISONIAZID (*Nydrazid*, others)
Occasional: peripheral neuropathy; liver damage, potentially fatal, particularly in patients more than 35 years old; glossitis and GI disturbance; allergic reactions; fever
Rare: blood dyscrasias; red cell aplasia; depression; agitation; auditory and visual hallucinations; paranoia; optic neuritis; hyperglycemia; folate and vitamin B_6 deficiency; pellagra-like rash; keratitis; lupus erythematosus-like syndrome; chronic liver injury; cirrhosis; Stevens-Johnson syndrome

ITRACONAZOLE *(Sporanox)*
Occasional: nausea; epigastric pain; headache; dizziness; edema; hypokalemia; rash; hepatic toxicity
Rare: congestive heart failure

IVERMECTIN *(Stromectol)*
Occasional: Mazzotti-type reaction seen in onchocerciasis, including fever, pruritus, tender lymph nodes, headache, and joint and bone pain
Rare: hypotension

KANAMYCIN (*Kantrex*, others)
Occasional: eighth-nerve damage affecting mainly hearing that may be irreversible and may not be detected until after therapy has been stopped (most likely with renal impairment); renal damage
Rare: rash; fever; peripheral neuritis; parenteral or intraperitoneal administration may produce neuromuscular blockade and apnea, not reversed by neostigmine or calcium gluconate

KETOCONAZOLE *(Nizoral)*
Frequent: nausea; vomiting
Occasional: decreased testosterone synthesis; gynecomastia; oligospermia and impotence in men; abdominal pain; rash; hepatitis; pruritus; dizziness; constipation; diarrhea; fever and chills; photophobia; headache
Rare: fatal hepatic necrosis; liver injury with jaundice; transient elevated transaminase; severe epigastric burning and pain; may interfere with adrenal function; anaphylaxis

LAMIVUDINE (3TC; *Epivir*)
Rare: headache; nausea; dizziness; nasal symptoms; rash; pancreatitis in children; neuropathy; lactic acidosis

LEVOFLOXACIN — See Fluoroquinolones

LINCOMYCIN (*Lincocin*, others)
Frequent: diarrhea, sometimes progressing to severe pseudomembranous colitis
Occasional: allergic reactions, rarely anaphylactic
Rare: blood dyscrasias; hypotension with rapid IV injection

LINEZOLID *(Zyvox)*
Frequent: GI disturbance; thrombocytopenia particularly with treatment greater than 2 weeks; anemia; myelosuppression; increased aminotransferase activity

LOMEFLOXACIN — See Fluoroquinolones

LOPINAVIR/RITONAVIR *(Kaletra)*
Similar to ritonavir, but less common; nephrotoxicity has not been reported
Rare: pancreatitis, may be fatal

LORACARBEF — See Cephalosporins

MALATHION *(Ovide)*
Occasional: local irritation

MEBENDAZOLE *(Vermox)*
Occasional: diarrhea; abdominal pain; migration of ascaris through mouth and nose
Rare: leukopenia; agranulocytosis; hypospermia

MEFLOQUINE *(Lariam)*
Frequent: vertigo; lightheadedness; nausea, other GI disturbances; nightmares; visual disturbances; headache; insomnia
Occasional: confusion
Rare: psychosis; hypotension; convulsions; coma; paresthesias

MEGLUMINE ANTIMONIATE *(Glucantime)* — Similar to sodium stibogluconate

MELARSOPROL *(Mel B)*
Frequent: myocardial damage; albuminuria; hypertension; colic; Herxheimer-type reaction; encephalopathy; vomiting; peripheral neuropathy
Rare: shock

MEROPENEM *(Merrem)* — Similar to imipenem, but may be less likely to cause seizures

METHENAMINE MANDELATE (*Mandelamine*, others) and **METHENAMINE HIPPURATE** *(Hiprex, Urex)*
Occasional: GI disturbance; dysuria; allergic reactions

METHICILLIN — See Penicillins

METRONIDAZOLE (*Flagyl*, others)
Frequent: nausea; headache; anorexia; metallic taste
Occasional: vomiting; diarrhea; insomnia; weakness; dry mouth; stomatitis; vertigo; tinnitus; paresthesias; rash; dark urine; urethral burning; disulfiram-like reaction with alcohol; candidiasis
Rare: pseudomembranous colitis; leukopenia; pancreatitis; seizures; peripheral neuropathy; encephalopathy; cerebellar syndrome with ataxia, dysarthria and MRI abnormalities

MICONAZOLE *(Monistat)*
Occasional: phlebitis; thrombocytosis; chills; intense, persistent pruritus; rash; vomiting; hyperlipidemia; dizziness; blurred vision; local burning and irritation with topical use
Rare: anemia; thrombocytopenia; hyponatremia; renal insufficiency; anaphylaxis; cardiac and respiratory arrest with initial dose

MINOCYCLINE — See Tetracyclines

MOXIFLOXACIN — See Fluoroquinolones

NAFCILLIN — See Penicillins

NALIDIXIC ACID (*NegGram*, others)
Frequent: GI disturbance; rash; visual disturbance
Occasional: CNS disturbance; acute intracranial hypertension in young children and rarely in adults; photosensitivity reactions, sometimes persistent; convulsions; hyperglycemia
Rare: cholestatic jaundice; blood dyscrasias; fatal immune hemolytic anemia; arthralgia or arthritis; lupus-like syndrome; confusion, depression, excitement, visual hallucinations

NELFINAVIR *(Viracept)*
Frequent: mild to moderate diarrhea
Occasional: increased aminotransferase activity; rash; nausea; glucose intolerance; increased bleeding in hemophiliacs; hyperlipidemia; abnormal fat distribuation

NEOMYCIN
Occasional: eighth-nerve and renal damage, same as with kanamycin but hearing loss may be more frequent and severe and may occur with oral, intra-articular, irrigant, or topical use; GI disturbance; malabsorption with oral use; contact dermatitis with topical use
Rare: neuromuscular blockade and apnea that may be reversed by intravenous neostigmine or calcium gluconate; pseudomembranous colitis

NEVIRAPINE *(Viramune)*
Frequent: rash, can progress to Stevens-Johnson syndrome
Occasional: fever; nausea; headache; hepatotoxicity, which can be fatal

NICLOSAMIDE *(Niclocide)*
Occasional: nausea; abdominal pain

NIFURTIMOX *(Lampit)*
Frequent: anorexia; vomiting; weight loss; loss of memory; sleep disorders; tremor; paresthesias; weakness; polyneuritis
Rare: convulsions; fever; pulmonary infiltrates and pleural effusion

NITROFURANTOIN (*Macrodantin*, others)
Frequent: GI disturbance; allergic reactions, including pulmonary infiltrates
Occasional: lupus-like syndrome; blood dyscrasias; hemolytic anemia; peripheral neuropathy, sometimes severe; pulmonary fibrosis
Rare: cholestatic jaundice; chronic active hepatitis, sometimes fatal; focal nodular hyperplasia of liver; pancreatitis; trigeminal neuralgia; crystalluria; increased intracranial pressure; lactic acidosis; parotitis; severe hemolytic anemia in G-6-PD deficiency

NORFLOXACIN — See Fluoroquinolones

NYSTATIN (*Mycostatin*, others)
Occasional: allergic reactions; fixed drug eruption; GI disturbance

OFLOXACIN — See Fluoroquinolones

ORNIDAZOLE *(Tiberal)*
Occasional: dizziness; headache; GI disturbance
Rare: reversible peripheral neuropathy

OSELTAMIVIR PHOSPHATE *(TamiFlu)*
Occasional: nausea; vomiting; headache

OXACILLIN — See Penicillins

OXAMNIQUINE *(Vansil)*
Occasional: headache; fever; dizziness; somnolence and insomnia; nausea; diarrhea; rash; increased aminotransferase activity; ECG changes; EEG changes; orange-red discoloration of urine
Rare: seizures; neuropsychiatric disturbances

OXYTETRACYCLINE — See Tetracyclines

PARA-AMINOSALICYLIC ACID — See Aminosalicylic acid

PAROMOMYCIN (aminosidine; *Humatin*)
Frequent: GI disturbance with oral use
Rare: eighth-nerve damage (mainly auditory) and renal damage when aminosidine is given IV; vertigo; pancreatitis

PENICILLINS
(amoxicillin – *Amoxil*, others; amoxicillin/clavulanic acid – *Augmentin*; ampicillin – *Principen*, others; ampicillin/sulbactam – *Unasyn*; carbenicillin indanyl – *Geocillin*; cloxacillin; dicloxacillin – *Dycill*, others; methicillin; mezlocillin – *Mezlin*; nafcillin – *Nafcil*, others; oxacillin; penicillin G; penicillin V; piperacillin – *Pipracil*; piperacillin/ tazobactam – *Zosyn*; ticarcillin – *Ticar*; ticarcillin/clavulanic acid – *Timentin*)
Frequent: allergic reactions, rarely anaphylaxis, erythema multiforme or Stevens Johnson syndrome; rash (more common with ampicillin and amoxicillin than with other penicillins); diarrhea (most common with ampicillin and amoxicillin/clavulanic acid); nausea and vomiting with amoxicillin/clavulanic acid in children
Occasional: hemolytic anemia; neutropenia; pseudomembranous colitis; platelet dysfunction with high doses of piperacillin, ticarcillin, nafcillin, or methicillin; cholestatic heptiis with amoxicillin/clavulanic acid
Rare: hepatic damage with semisynthetic penicillins; granulocytopenia or agranulocytosis with semisynthetic penicillins; renal damage with semisynthetic penicillins and penicillin G; muscle irritability and seizures, usually after high doses in patients with impaired renal function; hyperkalemia and arrhythmias with IV potassium penicillin G given rapidly; bleeding diathesis; Henoch-Schönlein purpura with ampicillin; thrombocytopenia with methicillin and mezlocillin; terror, hallucinations, disorientation, agitation, bizarre behavior and neurological reactions with high doses of procaine penicillin G, oxacillin, or ticarcillin; hypokalemic alkalosis and/or sodium overload with high doses of ticarcillin or nafcillin; hemorrhagic cystitis with methicillin; GI bleeding with dicloxacillin; tissue damage with extravasation of nafcillin

PENTAMIDINE ISETHIONATE (*Pentam 300, NebuPent*, others)
Frequent: hypotension; hypoglycemia often followed by diabetes mellitus; vomiting; blood dyscrasias; renal damage; pain at injection site; GI disturbance
Occasional: may aggravate diabetes; shock; hypocalcemia; liver damage; cardiotoxicity; delirium; rash
Rare: Herxheimer-type reaction; anaphylaxis; acute pancreatitis; hyperkalemia

PERMETHRIN (*Nix* others)
Occasional: burning; stinging; numbness; increased pruritus; pain; edema; erythema; rash

PIPERACILLIN — See Penicillins

PIPERACILLIN/TAZOBACTAM — See Penicillins

POLYMYXINS
(colistimethate – *Coly-Mycin*, polymyxin B – generic)
Occasional: renal damage; peripheral neuropathy; thrombophlebitis at IV injection site with polymyxin B
Rare: allergic reactions; neuromuscular blockade and apnea with parenteral administration, not reversed by neostigmine but may be by IV calcium chloride

PRAZIQUANTEL *(Biltricide)*
Frequent: abdominal pain; diarrhea; malaise; headache; dizziness
Occasional: sedation; fever; sweating; nausea; eosinophilia
Rare: pruritus; rash; edema; hiccups

PRIMAQUINE PHOSPHATE
Frequent: hemolytic anemia in G-6-PD deficiency
Occasional: neutropenia; GI disturbance; methemoglobinemia
Rare: CNS symptoms; hypertension; arrhythmias

PROGUANIL *(Paludrine; Malarone* [with atovaquone])
Occasional: oral ulceration; hair loss; scaling of palms and soles; urticaria
Rare: hematuria (with large doses); vomiting; abdominal pain; diarrhea (with large doses); thrombocytopenia

PYRANTEL PAMOATE (*Antiminth*, others)
Occasional: GI disturbance; headache; dizziness; rash; fever

PYRAZINAMIDE
Frequent: arthralgia; hyperuricemia
Occasional: liver damage; GI disturbance; acute gouty arthritis; rash
Rare: photosensitivity reactions; acute hypertension

PYRETHRINS with PIPERONYL BUTOXIDE (*RID*, others)
Occasional: allergic reactions

PYRIMETHAMINE *(Daraprim)*
Occasional: blood dyscrasias; folic acid deficiency
Rare: rash; vomiting; convulsions; shock; possibly pulmonary eosinophilia; fatal cutaneous reactions with **pyrimethamine-sulfadoxine** *(Fansidar)*

QUINACRINE
Frequent: disulfiram-like reaction with alcohol; nausea and vomiting; colors skin and urine yellow
Occasional: headache; dizziness
Rare: rash; fever; psychosis; extensive exfoliative dermatitis in patients with psoriasis

QUININE SULFATE — See Quinine Dihydrochloride

QUININE DIHYDROCHLORIDE
Frequent: cinchonism (tinnitus, headache, nausea, abdominal pain, visual disturbance)
Occasional: deafness; hemolytic anemia; other blood dyscrasias; photosensitivity reactions; hypoglycemia; arrhythmias; hypotension; fever
Rare: blindness; sudden death if injected too rapidly; hypersensitivity reaction with TTP-HUS

QUINUPRISTIN/DALFOPRISTIN *(Synercid)*
Frequent: local irritation and thrombophlebitis with peripheral IV administration; arthralgias; myalgias; increase in conjugated bilirubin
Occasional: nausea; rash; increased aminotransferase activity

RIBAVIRIN *(Virazole, Rebetron* with interferon alfa)
Occasional: anemia; headache; abdominal cramps and nausea; fatigue; elevation of bilirubin; teratogenic and embryolethal in animals and mutagenic in mammalian cells; rash; conjunctivitis; bronchospasm with aerosol use; hyperuricemia; depression

RIFABUTIN *(Mycobutin)* — Similar to rifampin; also iritis, uveitis, leukopenia, arthralgia

RIFAMPIN *(Rifadin, Rimactane)*
Frequent: colors urine, tears, saliva, CSF, contact lenses, and lens implants red-orange
Occasional: liver damage; GI disturbance; allergic reactions
Rare: flu-like syndrome, sometimes with thrombocytopenia, hemolytic anemia, shock, and renal failure, particularly with intermittent therapy; acute organic brain syndrome; acute adrenal crisis in patients with adrenal insufficiency; renal damage; severe proximal myopathy

RIFAMPIN-ISONIAZID *(Rifamate)* — See individual drugs

RIFAMPIN-ISONIAZID-PYRAZINAMIDE *(Rifater)* — See individual drugs

RIFAPENTINE *(Priftin)* — Similar to rifampin; higher rate of hyperuricemia

RIMANTADINE *(Flumadine)* — Similar to amantadine, but lower risk of CNS effects

RITONAVIR *(Norvir)*
Frequent: nausea; diarrhea; vomiting; asthenia; elevated serum triglycerides, cholesterol
Occasional: abdominal pain; anorexia; dyspepsia; circumoral and peripheral paresthesias; rash; altered taste; increased aminotransferase activity; cholestasis; glucose intolerance; abnormal fat distribution; increased bleeding in hemophiliacs
Rare: nephrotoxicity; hyperprolactinemia

SAQUINAVIR *(Invirase; Fortovase)*
Occasional: diarrhea; abdominal discomfort; nausea; glucose intolerance; hyperlipidemia; abnormal fat distribution; increased aminotransferase activity; increased bleeding in hemophiliacs
Rare: rash; hyperprolactinemia

SODIUM STIBOGLUCONATE *(Pentostam)*
Frequent: muscle and joint pain; fatigue; nausea; increased aminotransferase activity; T-wave flattening or inversion; pancreatitis
Occasional: weakness; abdominal pain; liver damage; bradycardia; leukopenia; thrombocytopenia; rash; vomiting
Rare: diarrhea; pruritus; myocardial damage; hemolytic anemia; renal damage; shock; sudden death

SPECTINOMYCIN *(Trobicin)*
Occasional: soreness at injection site; urticaria; dizziness; nausea; chills; fever; insomnia; decreased urine output; allergic reactions

SPIRAMYCIN *(Rovamycine)*
Occasional: GI disturbance
Rare: allergic reactions

STAVUDINE (D4T; *Zerit)*
Frequent: peripheral neuropathy
Occasional: increased aminotransferase activity; lactic acidosis; loss of subcutaneous fat
Rare: rash; pancreatitis

STREPTOMYCIN
Frequent: eighth-nerve damage (mainly vestibular), sometimes permanent; paresthesias; rash; fever; eosinophilia
Occasional: pruritus; anaphylaxis; renal damage
Rare: blood dyscrasias; neuromuscular blockade and apnea with parenteral administration, usually reversed by neostigmine; optic neuritis; hepatic necrosis; myocarditis; hemolytic anemia; renal failure; pseudomembranous colitis; toxic erythema; Stevens-Johnson syndrome

SULFONAMIDES
Frequent: allergic reactions (rash, photosensitivity, drug fever)
Occasional: kernicterus in newborn; renal damage; liver damage; Stevens-Johnson syndrome (particularly with long-acting sulfonamides); hemolytic anemia; other blood dyscrasias; vasculitis
Rare: transient acute myopia; pseudomembranous colitis; reversible infertility in men with sulfasalazine; CNS toxicity with trimethoprim-sulfamethoxazole in patients with AIDS

SURAMIN SODIUM
Frequent: vomiting; pruritus; urticaria; paresthesias; hyperesthesia of hands and feet; peripheral neuropathy; photophobia
Occasional: kidney damage; blood dyscrasias; shock; optic atrophy

TENOFOVIR *(Viread)*
Occasional: diarrhea; nausea; vomiting; flatulence

TERBINAFINE *(Lamisil)*
Frequent: headache; GI disturbance
Occasional: Taste disturbance; rash; pruritus; urticaria; toxic epidermal necrolysis; erythema multiforme; increased aminotransferase activity
Rare: serious hepatic injury; anaphylaxis; pancytopenia; agranulocytosis; severe neutropenia; changes in ocular lens and retina; parotid swelling; congestive heart failure

TETRACYCLINES
(demeclocycline – *Declomycin*; doxycycline – *Vibramycin*, others; minocycline – *Minocin*, others; oxytetracycline – *Terramycin*, others; tetracycline hydrochloride – *Sumycin*, others)
Frequent: GI disturbance; bone lesions and staining and deformity of teeth in children up to 8 years old, and in the newborn when given to pregnant women after the fourth month of pregnancy
Occasional: malabsorption; enterocolitis; photosensitivity reactions (most frequent with demeclocycline); vestibular toxicity with minocycline; increased azotemia with renal insufficiency (except doxycycline, but exacerbation of renal failure with doxycycline has been reported); renal insufficiency with demeclocycline in cirrhotic patients; hepatic injury; parenteral doses may cause serious liver damage, especially in pregnant women and patients with renal disease receiving 1 gram or more daily; esophageal

ulcerations; cutaneous and mucosal hyperpigmentation, tooth discoloration in adults with minocycline
Rare: allergic reactions, including serum sickness and anaphylaxis; pseudomembranous colitis; blood dyscrasias; drug-induced lupus with minocycline; auto-immune hepatitis; increased intracranial pressure; fixed-drug eruptions; diabetes insipidus with demeclocycline; transient acute myopia; blurred vision, diplopia, papilledema; photo-onycholysis and onycholysis; acute interstitial nephritis with minocycline; aggravation of myasthenic symptoms with IV injection, reversed with calcium; possibly transient neuropathy; hemolytic anemia

THIABENDAZOLE *(Mintezol)*
Frequent: nausea; vomiting; vertigo; headache; drowsiness; pruritus
Occasional: leukopenia; crystalluria; rash; hallucinations and other psychiatric reactions; visual and olfactory disturbance; erythema multiforme
Rare: shock; tinnitus; intrahepatic cholestasis; convulsions; angioneurotic edema; Stevens-Johnson syndrome

TICARCILLIN — See Penicillins

TICARCILLIN/CLAVULANIC ACID — See Penicillins

TINIDAZOLE *(Fasigyn)*
Occasional: metallic taste; nausea and vomiting; rash

TOBRAMYCIN (*Nebcin*, others) — Similar to gentamicin
Rare: delirium

TRIFLURIDINE *(Viroptic)*
Occasional: burning or stinging; palpebral edema
Rare: epithelial keratopathy; hypersensitivity reactions

TRIMETHOPRIM (*Proloprim*, others)
Frequent: nausea, vomiting with high doses
Occasional: megaloblastic anemia; thrombocytopenia; neutropenia; rash; fixed drug eruption
Rare: pancytopenia; hyperkalemia

TRIMETHOPRIM/SULFAMETHOXAZOLE (*Bactrim, Septra*, others)
Frequent: rash; fever; nausea and vomiting
Occasional: hemolysis in G-6-PD deficiency; acute megaloblastic anemia; granulocytopenia; thrombocytopenia; pseudomembranous colitis; kernicterus in newborn; hyperkalemia
Rare: agranulocytosis; aplastic anemia; hepatotoxicity; Stevens-Johnson syndrome; aseptic meningitis; fever; confusion; depression; hallucinations; deterioration in renal disease; intrahepatic cholestasis; methemoglobinemia; pancreatitis; ataxia; CNS toxicity in patients with AIDS; renal tubular acidosis; hyperkalemia

TRIMETREXATE (*Neutrexin;* with "leucovorin rescue")
Occasional: rash; peripheral neuropathy; bone marrow depression; increased serum aminotransferase activity

TROLEANDOMYCIN *(TAO)*
Occasional: stomatitis; GI disturbance; cholestatic jaundice
Rare: allergic reactions

VALACYCLOVIR *(Valtrex)* — Generally same as acyclovir
Rare: thrombotic thrombocytopenic purpura/hemolytic uremic syndrome in severely immunocompromised patients treated with high doses

VALGANCICLOVIR *(Valcyte)* — Generally same as ganciclovir

VANCOMYCIN (*Vancocin*, others)
Frequent: thrombophlebitis; fever, chills
Occasional: eighth-nerve damage (mainly hearing) especially with large or continued doses (more than 10 days), in presence of renal damage, and in the elderly; neutropenia; renal damage; allergic reactions; rash; "redman" syndrome
Rare: peripheral neuropathy; hypotension with rapid IV administration; exfoliative dermatitis

VORICONAZOLE *(Vfend)*
Frequent: transient visual disturbances
Occasional: rash; increased aminotransferase activity
Rare: photosensitivity with prolonged use

ZALCITABINE (ddC; *Hivid*)
Frequent: peripheral neuropathy
Occasional: stomatitis; esophageal ulceration; nausea; headache; fever; fatigue; abdominal pain; diarrhea; rash
Rare: pancreatitis; hypersensitivity reaction with fever, GI or respiratory symptoms and rash

ZANAMIVIR *(Relenza)*
Occasional: nasal and throat discomfort; headache; cough; bronchospasm in patients with asthma

ZIDOVUDINE *(Retrovir)*
Frequent: anemia; granulocytopenia; nail pigment changes; nausea; fatigue
Occasional: headache; insomnia; confusion; diarrhea; rash; fever; myalgias; myopathy; light-headedness; lactic acidosis
Rare: seizures; Wernicke's encephalopathy; cholestatic hepatitis; transient ataxia and nystagmus with acute large overdosage

DOSAGE OF ANTIMICROBIAL AGENTS

In choosing the dosage of an antimicrobial drug, the physician must consider the site of infection, the identity and antimicrobial susceptibility of the infecting organism, the possible toxicity of the drug of choice, and the condition of the patient, with special attention to renal function. This article and the table that follows on page 162 offer some guidelines for determining antimicrobial dosage, but dosage recommendations taken out of context of the clinical situation may be misleading.

RENAL INSUFFICIENCY — Antimicrobial drugs excreted through the urinary tract may be toxic for patients with renal insufficiency if they are given in usual therapeutic doses, because serum concentrations in these patients may become dangerously high. Nephrotoxic and ototoxic drugs such as gentamicin or other aminoglycosides may damage the kidney, further decreasing the excretion of these drugs, leading to higher blood concentrations that may be ototoxic and may cause additional renal damage. In patients with renal insufficiency, therefore, an antimicrobial drug with minimal nephrotoxicity, such as a beta-lactam, is preferred. When nephrotoxic drugs must be used, renal function should be monitored. Measurements of serum creatinine or blood urea nitrogen (BUN) concentrations are useful as indices of renal function, but are not as accurate as measurements of creatinine clearance; serum creatinine and BUN concentrations may be normal even with significant loss of renal function.

In renal insufficiency, control of serum concentrations of potentially toxic drugs can be achieved either by varying the dose or by varying the interval between doses. Serum antimicrobial concentrations should be measured whenever possible; rigid adherence to any dosage regimen can result in either inadequate or toxic serum concentrations in patients with renal insufficiency, particularly when renal function is changing rapidly.

CHILDREN'S DOSAGE — Many antimicrobial drugs have such a broad therapeutic index that it makes no difference in practice if children's dosage is based on weight or on surface area. Where dosage considerations are important in preventing severe toxic effects, as with the aminoglycosides, recommendations for safe usage are derived primarily from experience with dosage based on weight.

ONCE-DAILY AMINOGLYCOSIDES — Current data suggest that in certain categories of patients once-daily doses of gentamicin, tobramycin and amikacin are as effective for many indications as multiple daily doses and are equally or less nephrotoxic (TC Bailey et al, Clin Infect Dis 1997; 24:786; CD Freeman, J Antimicrob Chemother 1997; 39:677). Monitoring 24-hour trough drug levels is recommended to minimize the risk of toxicity. Once-daily doses of aminoglycosides are not recommended for treatment of endocarditis and should be used cautiously in the elderly, immunocompromised patients and those with renal insufficiency.

THE TABLE — Dosage – The recommendations in the table that follows are based on the judgment of Medical Letter consultants. In some cases they differ from the manufacturer's recommendations, partly because clinical experience reported after the labeling is approved is not always reflected by an appropriate change in the manufacturer's recommendations. The range of dosage specified for some drugs may not include relatively rare indications. In general, lower doses are sufficient for treatment of urinary tract infection, and higher doses are recommended for such severe infections as meningitis, endocarditis and the sepsis syndrome.

Interval – More than one interval between doses is recommended for some drugs. In general, the longer intervals should be used for infections of the urinary tract and for intramuscular administration. Recommendations are made in hours, but many oral drugs can be given three or four times during the daytime for convenience. For maximum absorption, which is often not necessary, most oral antibiotics should be given at least 30 minutes before or two hours after a meal.

ANTIMICROBIAL DRUG DOSAGE†

	ADULTS		CHILDREN	
	ORAL	PARENTERAL	ORAL	PARENTERAL
Abacavir	300 mg q12h		8 mg/kg q12h	
Acyclovir	200 mg q4h x 5 or 400 mg q8h[1]	5-15 mg/kg q8h	20 mg/kg q6h	5-20 mg/kg q8h
Amantadine	100 mg q12-24h		4.4 mg/kg q12-24h	
Amikacin		5 mg/kg q8h, 7.5 mg/kg q12h or 15 mg/kg q24h		5 mg/kg q8h or 7.5 mg/kg q12h
Amoxicillin	250-500 mg q8h or 500-875 mg q12h		6.6-13.3 mg/kg q8h or 15 mg/kg q12h	
Amoxicillin/ clavulanic acid	250-500 mg[3] q8h or 500-875 mg[3] q12h		6.6-13.3 mg/kg[3] q8h or 15 mg/kg[3] q12h	
Amphotericin B		0.3-1.5 mg/kg[4] q24h		0.3-1.5 mg/kg[4] q24h
Amphotericin B cholesteryl sulfate complex		3-4 mg/kg q24h		3-4 mg/kg q24h
Amphotericin B lipid complex		5 mg/kg q24h		5 mg/kg q24h
Amphotericin B liposomal		3-5 mg/kg q24h		3-5 mg/kg q24h
Ampicillin	500 mg q6h	1-2 g q4-6h	12.5-25 mg/kg q6h	25-50 mg/kg q6h[7]
Ampicillin/ sulbactam		1.5-3 g[8] q6h		50 mg/kg[8] q6h

† Antiparasitic drug dosages are found in the article on this subject. The articles on antiviral and antifungal drugs, prophylaxis, sexually transmitted diseases and HIV infection also include dosage recommendations.

1. For treatment of initial genital herpes. For suppression of genital herpes, 400 mg q12h is used. For treatment of varicella, 800 mg q6h and for zoster 800 mg 5 times daily every 4 hours are recommended.
2. Give full dose once, then monitor levels.
3. Dosage based on amoxicillin content. For doses of 500 or 875 mg, 500-mg or 875-mg tablets should be used, because multiple smaller tablets would contain too much clavulanic acid. The 875-mg, 500-mg and 250-mg tablets each contain 125 mg clavulanic acid. 125-mg chewable tablets and 125 mg/5 ml oral suspension both contain 31.25 mg clavulanic acid; 250-mg chewable tablets and 250-mg/5-ml oral suspension both contain 62.5 mg clavulanic acid.

USUAL MAXIMUM DOSE/DAY	ADULT DOSAGE IN RENAL FAILURE				Extra Dose After Hemodialysis
		For Creatinine Clearance (ml/min)			
	Dose	80-50	50-10	<10	
600 mg	Not recommended				
4 g oral 45 mg/kg IV	10 mg/kg	q8h	q12-24h	2.5 mg/kg q24h	yes
200 mg		100 mg q24h	100-200 mg q24-48h	200 mg q7d	no
1.5 g	5 mg/kg	q12h	q24-36h	See foot-note 2	yes
3 g	500 mg	q8h	q12h	q24h	yes
1.5 g	500 mg[3]	q8h	q12h	q24h	yes
1 mg/kg[5]	Change not required[6]				no
4 mg/kg	Unknown				
5 mg/kg	Unknown				
5 mg/kg	Unknown				
14 g	0.5-2 g	q6h	q8h	q12h	yes
12g	1.5-3 g[8]	no change	q8-12h	q24h	yes

4. Given IV once a day, over a period of two to four hours.
5. Or up to 1.5 mg/kg given every other day.
6. Amphotericin B is potentially nephrotoxic. A pre- and post-dose IV bolus of 500 ml normal saline may decrease toxicity. Temporary interruption of therapy may be required when the serum creatinine exceeds 3 mg/dl.
7. For meningitis in children caused by ampicillin-sensitive *H. influenzae* type b, Medical Letter consultants recommend up to 400 mg/kg/day. Meningitis should be treated q4h.
8. Combination formulation: 1.5-g vial contains 1 g ampicillin/500 mg sulbactam; 3-g vial contains 2 g ampicillin/1 g sulbactam.

	ADULTS		CHILDREN	
	ORAL	PARENTERAL	ORAL	PARENTERAL
Amprenavir[9]	1200 mg q12h		20 mg/kg q12h[10] or 15 mg/kg q8h[10]	
Azithromycin	250-1000 mg[11] q24h	500 mg q24h	5-12 mg/kg[11] q24h	
Aztreonam[9]		1-2 g q6-8h		30 mg/kg q6-8h
Carbenicillin indanyl sodium	1-2 tablets[12] q6h		7.5-12.5 mg/kg q12h	
Caspofungin		70 mg day 1, then 50 mg q24h[13,14]		See footnote 14
Cefaclor	250-500 mg q8h or 375-500 mg q12h		6.6-13.3 mg/kg q8h	
Cefadroxil	1 g q12-24h		15 mg/kg q12h	
Cefamandole		500 mg-2 g q4-8h		50-150 mg/kg/day, divided q4-8h
Cefazolin		500 mg-1.5 g q6-8h		25-100 mg/kg/day, divided q6-8h
Cefdinir	300 mg q12h or 600 mg q24h		7 mg/kg q12h or 14 mg/kg q24h	
Cefditoren pivoxil	200-400 mg q12h		See footnote 15	
Cefepime		1-2 g q8-12h		50 mg/kg q8-12h
Cefixime	200 mg q12h or 400 mg q24h		4 mg/kg q12h or 8 mg/kg q24h	
Cefonicid		500 mg-2 g q24h		
Cefoperazone[9]		500 mg-4 g q6-12h		25-100 mg/kg q12h

9. Dosage adjustment may be necessary in patients with hepatic dysfunction.
10. Using capsules. Also available in solution: 22.5 mg/kg q12h or 17 mg/kg q8h (max. 2800 mg/day).
11. For adults: 500 mg on day 1 and 250 mg/day on days 2-5; urethritis and cervicitis: 1 g once for *C. trachomatis*, 2 g once for *N. gonorrhoeae*. For children: pharyngitis/tonsillitis: 12 mg/kg once a day for 5 days; acute otitis media: 10 mg/kg on day 1 and 5 mg/kg on days 2 to 5 or single-dose 30 mg/kg or 10 mg/kg once daily for 3 days.
12. Tablets contain 382 mg of carbenicillin.

USUAL MAXIMUM DOSE/DAY	ADULT DOSAGE IN RENAL FAILURE				
		For Creatinine Clearance (ml/min)			Extra Dose After Hemodialysis
	Dose	80-50	50-10	<10	
2400 mg/day	Change not required				
500 mg	Change not required				
8 g		500-1000 mg q8h	500-750 mg q8h	250-500 mg q8h	yes
3 g	See package insert				
50 mg	Change not required				no
4 g	Change not required				yes
2 g	500 mg	q12-24h	q12-24h	q36h	yes
12 g		1-2 g q6h	1-2 g q8h	0.5-1 g q8-12h	yes
6 g		1 g q8h	1 g q8-12h	1 g q24h	yes
600 mg	300 mg	No change	q24h	q24h	yes
800 mg	200-400 mg	No change	200 mg q12-24h	Unknown	
6 g	2 g	q12h	1-2 g q24h	500 mg q24h	yes
400 mg	200-400 mg	q24h	q24h	200 mg q24h	no
2 g		0.5-1.5 g q24h	0.25-1 g q24-48h	0.25-1 g q3-5 days	no
12 g	Change not required				no*

* But give usual dose after dialysis.

13. For patients with moderate hepatic insufficiency (Child-Pugh score 7-9) the daily dose should be reduced to 35 mg following the standard 70 mg loading dose on day 1.
14. Not approved for use in children. Limited experience in clinical trials with 1 mg/kg q24h.
15. Has not been studied in children.

	ADULTS		CHILDREN	
	ORAL	PARENTERAL	ORAL	PARENTERAL
Cefotaxime		1-2 g q4-12h		50-180 mg/kg/day divided q4-6h
Cefotetan		500 mg-3 g q12h		
Cefoxitin		1-3 g q4-6h		80-160 mg/kg/day, divided q4-6h
Cefpodoxime	100-400 mg q12h		10 mg/kg q24h or 5 mg/kg q12h	
Cefprozil	250-500 mg q12h		15 mg/kg q12h	
Ceftazidime		250 mg-2 g q8-12h		30-50 mg/kg q8h
Ceftibuten	400 mg q24h		9 mg/kg q24h	
Ceftizoxime		500 mg-4 g q8-12h		50 mg/kg q6-8h
Ceftriaxone		1-2 g q12-24h		50-100 mg/kg/day, divided q12-24h
Cefuroxime		750 mg-1.5 g q8h		50-150 mg/kg/day, divided q6-8h
Cefuroxime axetil	125-500 mg q12h		10-15 mg/kg q12h	
Cephalexin	250 mg-1 g q6h		6.25-25 mg/kg q6h	
Cephapirin		500 mg-2 g q4-6h		40-80 mg/kg/day, divided q4-6h
Cephradine	250 mg-1 g q6h or 500 mg-1 g q12h	500 mg-2 g q6h	6.25-25 mg/kg q6h or 12.5-50 mg/kg q12h	12.5-25 mg/kg q6h
Chloramphenicol[9]	12.5-25 mg/kg q6h	12.5-25 mg/kg[16] q6h	12.5-25 mg/kg q6h	12.5-25 mg/kg[16] q6h
Cidofovir		5 mg/kg once/wk x 2, then 5 mg/kg every other week		See footnote 15

16. IV administration; dosage should be adjusted according to serum concentration.

USUAL MAXIMUM DOSE/DAY	ADULT DOSAGE IN RENAL FAILURE	For Creatinine Clearance (ml/min)			Extra Dose After Hemodialysis
	Dose	80-50	50-10	<10	
12 g	1-2 g	No change	q6-12h	q12 24h	yes
6 g	1-3 g	q12h	q12-24h	q48h	yes
12 g		1-2 g q8h	1-2 g q12h	0.5-1 g q12-24h	yes
800 mg	200-400 mg	q12h	q24h	q24h	yes
1000 mg	250-500 mg	No change	q24h	q24h	yes
6 g	0.5-2 g	q8-12h	1 g q12-24h	0.5 g q24-48h	yes
400 mg		No change	100-200 mg q24h	100 mg q24h	no*
12 g		0.5-1.5 g q8h	0.25-1 g q12h	0.25-1 g q24-48h	yes
4 g			Change not required		no
9 g	0.75-1.5 g	q8h	q8-12h	q24h	yes
1 g			Change not required		yes
4 g	0.25-1 g	No change	q8-12h	q12-24h	yes
12 g	0.5-2 g	q6h	q8h	q12h	yes
8 g	1-2 g	q6h	q8h	q12-72h	yes
4 g			Change not required		no*
	5 mg/kg	No change	1-2 mg/kg	0.5 mg/kg	no

* But give usual dose after dialysis.

	ADULTS		CHILDREN	
	ORAL	PARENTERAL	ORAL	PARENTERAL
Cinoxacin	250 mg q6h or 500 mg q12h			
Ciprofloxacin	250-750 mg q12h	200-400 mg q12h		
Clarithromycin	250-500 mg q12h		7.5 mg/kg q12h	
Clindamycin[9]	150-450 mg q6h	150-900 mg q6-8h	2-8 mg/kg q6-8h	2.5-10 mg/kg q6h
Cloxacillin	500 mg-1g q6h		12.5-25 mg/kg q6h	
Cycloserine[17]	250-500 mg q12h		5-10 mg/kg q12h	
Delavirdine	400 mg tid			
Dicloxacillin	125-500 mg q6h		3.125 -6.25 mg/kg q6h	
Didanosine[18] (ddI)	60 kg:200 mg q12h or 400 mg q24h[18] <60 kg:125 mg q12h or 250 mg q24h[18]		90-120 mg/m^2 q12h[18]	
Dirithromycin	500 mg q24h		12 yrs: 500 mg q24h	
Doxycycline	100 mg q12-24h	100 mg q12-24h	2.2 mg/kg[19] q12-24h	2.2 mg/kg[19] q12-24h
Efavirenz	600 mg q24h		200-400 mg q24h	
Enoxacin	200-400 mg q12h		See foot-note 15	
Ertapenem sodium		1 gm q24h		Not recom-mended
Erythromycin	250-500 mg q6h	250 mg-1 g IV[21] q6h	7.5-12.5 mg/kg q6h	3.75-12.5 mg/kg IV[21] q6h

17. Monitor concentratons, toxicity increases markedly above 30 g/ml.
18. Refers to chewable, dispersible tablets. For adults and children more than one year old, each dose should include two tablets to supply adequate buffer. Didanosine also available in powder for oral solution for adults: 60 kg: 250 mg q12h, <60 kg: 167 mg q12h and as a delayed-release capsule for adults: 60 kg: 400 mg q24h, <60 kg: 250 q24h. A pediatric powder formulation is also available.

USUAL MAXIMUM DOSE/DAY	ADULT DOSAGE IN RENAL FAILURE				
	For Creatinine Clearance (ml/min)				Extra Dose After Hemodialysis
	Dose	80-50	50-10	<10	
1 g		250 mg q8h	250 mg q12-24h	250 mg q24h	no
1.5 g		No change	250-500 mg q12-18h	250-500 mg q24h	no*
1 g	250-500 mg	No change	q24h	Unknown	
4.8 g			Change not required		no
4 g			Change not required		no
1 g		No change	250 mg q12-24h	250 mg q24-48h	
1.2 g			Change not required		no
4 g			Change not required		no
400 mg		No change	100-200 mg q24h	75-100 mg q24h	yes
500 mg			Change not required		no
200 mg			Change not required		no
600 mg			Change not required		
800 mg	200-400 mg	No change	No change	q24h	no
1 g		No change	500 mg q24h	500 mg q24h	yes[20]
4 g			Change not required		no

* But give usual dose after dialysis.

19. Not recommended for children less than eight years old.
20. If the 500-mg dose is given 6 hours before hemodialysis, a supplemental dose of 150 mg is recommened after dialysis. If the 500-mg dose is given >6 hours before hemodialysis, no supplemental dose is needed.
21. By slow infusion to minimize thrombophlebitis.

	ADULTS		CHILDREN	
	ORAL	PARENTERAL	ORAL	PARENTERAL
Ethambutol[22]	15-25 mg/kg q24h		15-25 mg/kg q24h	
Ethionamide	250-500 mg q12h		7.5-10 mg/kg q12h	
Famciclovir	500 mg q8h[23]			
Fluconazole	50-400 mg q24h	100-400 mg q24h	3-12 mg/kg q24h	3-12 mg/kg q24h
Flucytosine	12.5-37.5 mg/kg q6h		12.5-37.5 mg/kg q6h	
Foscarnet		60 mg/kg q8h or 90 mg/kg q12h[25]		
Fosfomycin	3 g once			
Ganciclovir	1 g q8h	5 mg/kg[26] q12h		5 mg/kg[26] q12h
Gatifloxacin	200-400 mg q24h	200-400 mg q24h		
Gentamicin		1-2.5 mg/kg q8h or 5-7 mg/kg q24h		1-2.5 mg/kg q8h
Griseofulvin Microsize	500-1000 mg q24h		11 mg/kg q24h	
Ultra-microsize	330-660 mg q24h		7.25 mg/kg q24h	
Imipenem		250 mg-1 g[27] q6-8h		15-25 mg/kg[27] q6h
Indinavir[9]	800 mg q8h		350 mg/m^2 q8h	

22. Not recommended in children whose visual acuity cannot be monitored (<6 years old).
23. For herpes zoster. For first episode genital herpes, the dosage is 250 mg q8h. For genital herpes recurrence, it is 125 mg q12h. For suppression of genital herpes, it is 250 mg q12h.
24. If treatment is essential, begin with 15-25 mg/kg q24h and adjust daily dose to maintain the plasma concentration between 50 and 75 g/ml.

USUAL MAXIMUM DOSE/DAY	ADULT DOSAGE IN RENAL FAILURE For Creatinine Clearance (ml/min) Dose	80-50	50-10	<10	Extra Dose After Hemodialysis
2.5 g	20 mg/kg	No change	q24-36h	q48h	no*
1 g		No change	No change	500 mg q24h	no
1.5 g	500 mg	q12h	q24h	Not recom-mended	yes
400 mg	100-400 mg	No change	q48h	q72h	yes
150 mg/kg	12.5-37.5 mg/kg	No change	q12-24h	Not recom-mended[24]	yes
		40-50 mg/kg q12h[25]	50-60 mg/kg q24h[25]	Not recom-mended	yes
3 g	Change not required				
10 mg/kg		2.5 mg/kg[26] q12h	1.25-2.5 mg/kg[26] q24h	1.25 mg/kg[26] 3x/week	no*
	500-1000 mg PO	No change	500 mg once or q12h	500 mg 3x/week	no*
400 mg		No change	400 mg once, then 200 mg q24h	400 mg once, then 200 mg q24h	no*
7 mg/kg	1.5 mg/kg	q8-12h	q12-24h	See foot-note 2	yes
1 g	Change not required				
660 mg	Change not required				
4 g[28]	250-500 mg	q6-8h	q8-12h	q12h	yes
	Change not required				

* But give usual dose after dialysis.

25. For CMV, given over at least one hour for induction; for maintenance, 90-120 mg/kg daily over two hours. For HSV or VZV, 40 mg/kg q8h.
26. For CMV induction, give IV at constant rate over one hour; for maintenance without renal failure: 5 mg/kg 7 days/week or 6 mg/kg 5 days/week; for maintenance with renal failure: induction dose is reduced by half.
27. Doses are for imipenem, which is combined with equal weight of cilastatin as *Primaxin.*
28. Maximum dosage should be 4 g or 50 mg/kg, whichever is less.

	ADULTS		CHILDREN	
	ORAL	PARENTERAL	ORAL	PARENTERAL
Interferon alfa-2a, alfa-2b		3 MIU TIW SC or IM[29]		See foot-note 29
Pegylated, alfa-2b		1 g/kg SC q wk		
Isoniazid[9,30]	300 mg q24h		10-20 mg/kg q24h	
Itraconazole	100-200 mg q12-24h	200 mg q12h x 4, then 200 mg q24h	5 mg/kg q24h	
Kanamycin		5 mg/kg q8h or 7.5 mg/kg q12h		5 mg/kg/q8h or 7.5 mg/kg/q12h
Ketoconazole	200-400 mg q12-24h		3.3-6.6 mg/kg q24h	
Lamivudine	50 kg:150 mg q12h <50 kg:2 mg/kg q12h		4 mg/kg q12h	
Levofloxacin	250-750 mg q24h	250-750 mg q24h	See footnote 15	
Linezolid	400-600 mg q12h	600 mg q12h	See footnote 32	
Lomefloxacin	400 mg q24h			
Lopinavir/ Ritonavir	400 mg/ 100 mg q12h[33]		7-15 kg: 12/3 mg/kg q12h[33] 15-40 kg: 10/2.5 mg/kg q12h[33] >40 kg or 12 yrs: 400 mg/100 mg q12h[33]	
Loracarbef	200-400 mg q12h		7.5-15 mg/kg q12h	
Meropenem		1-2 g q8h		20-40 mg/kg q8h

29. For chronic hepatitis C in adults. For acute hepatitis C in adults the dosage is 5 MIU 24h x 3 weeks, then TIW. For chronic hepatitis B the dosage is 5 MIU 24h or 10 MIU TIW for adults and for children it is 3-6 MIU/m^2 TIW.
30. For prophylaxis of positive PPD in adults, 300 mg/d; in children, 10 mg/kg/d up to maximum of 300 mg.
31. IV itraconazole should not be used in patients with CrCl <30 ml/min.

USUAL MAXIMUM DOSE/DAY	ADULT DOSAGE IN RENAL FAILURE				
		For Creatinine Clearance (ml/min)			Extra Dose After Hemodialysis
	Dose	80-50	50-10	<10	
3 MIU	Change not required				
70 g		No change	Use caution		
300 mg	Change not required				no*
400 mg	Change not required; but see footnote 31				
1.5 g	5-7.5 mg/kg	q24h	q24-72h	See foot-note 2	yes
400 mg	Change not required				no
300 mg		No change	150 mg once then 100-150 mg/d	50-150 mg once then 25-50 mg/d	no
750 mg	500 mg	No change	500 mg once then 250 mg q24h	500 mg once then 250 mg q48h	no
1200 mg	Change not required				no*
400 mg		No change	400 mg once then 200 mg q24h	Unknown	no
800 mg/ 200 mg	Change not required				
800 mg	200-400 mg	No change	q24h	q3-5 days	yes
6 g		No change	0.5-1 g q12h	0.5 g q24h	

* But give usual dose after dialysis.

32. Not approved for use in children. Limited experience in clinical trials with 10 mg/kg q12h.
33. A dose increase is necesssary if coadministered with nevirapine or efavirenz in treatment-experienced patients when reduced susceptibility to lopinavir is suspected.

	ADULTS		CHILDREN	
	ORAL	PARENTERAL	ORAL	PARENTERAL
Methenamine hippurate[34]	1 g q12h		12.5-25 mg/kg q12h	
Methenamine mandelate[34]	1 g q6h		12.5-18.75 mg/kg q6h	
Metronidazole[9]	500 mg q6-8h[35]	500 mg q6-8h[35]	7.5 mg/kg q6-8h[35]	7.5 mg/kg q6-8h[35]
Miconazole[36]		600 mg-1.2 g q8h		6.6-13.3 mg/kg q8h
Moxifloxacin[9]	400 mg q24h	400 mg q24h	See footnote 15	
Nafcillin		500 mg-2 g q4-6h		25-50 mg/kg q6h
Nalidixic acid	1 g q6h		Not recommended	
Nelfinavir[9]	750 mg q8h or 1250 mg q12h		25-30 mg/kg q8h	
Nevirapine	200 mg/d x 14, followed by 200 mg bid		<8 yrs: 4 mg/kg/d x 14 followed by 7 mg/kg bid 8 yrs: 4 mg/kg/d x 14 followed by 4 mg/kg bid	
Nitrofurantoin	50-100 mg q6h	Not recommended	1.25-1.75 mg/kg q6h	Not recommended
Norfloxacin	400 mg q12h		See footnote 15	
Ofloxacin	200-400 mg q12h	200-400 mg q12h	See footnote 15	
Oseltamavir	75 mg q12h[37]		15 kg: 30 mg q12h 16-23 kg: 45 mg q12h 24-40 kg: 60 mg q12h >40 kg: 75 mg q12h	

34. Usually given with an acidifying agent.
35. Dosage for anaerobic bacterial infections. First dose should be 15 mg/kg loading dose. For antiparasitic dosages, see table beginning on page 120.

USUAL MAXIMUM DOSE/DAY	ADULT DOSAGE IN RENAL FAILURE				Extra Dose After Hemodialysis
	Dose	For Creatinine Clearance (ml/min) 80-50	50-10	<10	
4 g		No change	Not recommended		
4 g		No change	Not recommended		
4 g		Change not required			no*
3.6 g		Change not required			no
400 mg		Change not required			
12 g		Change not required			no
4 g		No change	No change	Not recom-mended	
2.5 g		Change not required			
400 mg		Unknown			
400 mg		No change	Not recommended		
800 mg	400 mg	No change	q12-24h	q24h	no
800 mg	200-400 mg	No change	q24h	100-200 mg q24h	no
150 mg	75 mg	No change	q24h	Not recom-mended	

36. The manufacturer recommends an initial test dose of 200 mg.
37. Dosage may be given once daily for influenza prophylaxis.

	ADULTS		CHILDREN	
	ORAL	PARENTERAL	ORAL	PARENTERAL
Oxacillin	500 mg-1 g q6h	500 mg-2 g q4-6h	12.5-25 mg/kg q6h	25-50 mg/kg q6h
Penicillin G[38]	250-500 mg q6h	1.2-24 million U/day, divided q2-12h[39]	6.25-12.5 mg/kg q6h	100,000-250,000 U/kg/day, divided q2-12h[39]
Penicillin V[38]	250-500 mg q6h		6.25-12.5 mg/kg q6h	
Piperacillin		3-4 g q4-6h		200-300 mg/kg/day, divided q4-6h
Piperacillin/tazobactam		3.375 g[41] q4-6h		240 mg/kg/day of piperacillin divided q8h
Pyrazinamide	15-30 mg/kg q24h		15-30 mg/kg q24h	
Quinupristin/dalfopristin		7.5 mg/kg q8-12h		See footnote 42
Ribavirin	75kg: 400 mg q AM and 600 mg q PM >75 kg 600 mg bid		Unknown	
Rifabutin	150 mg q12h or 300 mg q24h		See footnote 43	
Rifampin[9,44]	600 mg/day	600 mg/day	10-20 mg/kg/day	10-20 mg/kg/day
Rifapentine	600 mg once or twice weekly		Unknown	
Rimantadine[9]	100 mg once or q12h		5 mg/kg once	

38. One mg is equal to 1600 units.
39. The interval between parenteral doses can be as short as 2 hours for initial intravenous treatment of meningococcemia, or as long as 12 hours between intramuscular doses of penicillin G procaine.
40. Patients with severe renal insufficiency should be given no more than one third to one half the maximum daily dosage, i.e., instead of giving 24 million units per day, 10 million units could be given. Patients on lower doses usually tolerate full dosage even with severe renal insufficiency.

USUAL MAXIMUM DOSE/DAY	ADULT DOSAGE IN RENAL FAILURE For Creatinine Clearance (ml/min) Dose	80-50	50-10	<10	Extra Dose After Hemodialysis
12 g			Change not required		no
24 million units			Change not required; see footnote 40		yes
4 g			Change not required		yes
24 g	3-4 g	No change	q6-8h	q8-12h	yes
20.25 g	2.25-3.375 g[41]	No change	2.25 g[41] q6h	2.25 g[41] q8h	yes
2 g			Change not required		
Unknown			Change not required		
1200 mg		No change	Not recommended		
300 mg			Change not required		no
600 mg			Change not required		no
600 mg			Unknown		
200 mg			Change not required		no

41. Combination formulation: A 2.25-g vial contains 2 g piperacillin/250 mg tazobactam; a 3.375-g vial contains 3 g piperacillin/375 mg tazobactam; a 4.5-g vial contains 4 g piperacillin/500 mg tazobactam.
42. Safety has not been established, but quinupristin/dalfopristin 7.5 mg/kg q8-12h has been used in a limited number of children.
43. Safety has not been established, but rifabutin 5 mg/kg/d has been used in a limited number of children for treatment of *Mycobacterium avium* complex.
44. For meningococcal carriers, dosage is 600 mg bid x 2 days for adults, 10 mg/kg q12h x 2 days for children more than one month old, and 5 mg/kg q12h x 2 days for infants less than one month old.

	ADULTS		CHILDREN	
	ORAL	PARENTERAL	ORAL	PARENTERAL
Ritonavir[9]	600 mg q12h[45]		400 mg/m^2 q12h	
Saquinavir[46]	1200 mg q8h			
Spectinomycin		2 g once		40 mg/kg once
Stavudine[9]	60 kg: 40 mg q12h <60 kg: 30 mg q12h		30 kg: 30 mg q12h <30 kg: 1 mg/kg q12h	
Streptomycin		500 mg-1 g q12h		10-15 mg/kg q12h
Sulfisoxazole	500 mg-1 g q6h	25 mg/kg q6h	150 mg/kg/day divided q4-6h	100 mg/kg/day divided q6-8h
Tenofovir	300 mg q24h		See foot- note 15	
Tetracyclines[19,47]	250-500 mg q6h		6.25-12.5 mg/kg q6h	
Ticarcillin		200-300 mg/kg/day, divided q4-6h		200-300 mg/kg/day, divided q4-6h
Ticarcillin/ clavulanic acid		3.1 g[48] q4-6h		200-300 mg/kg/day,[48] divided q4-6h
Tobramycin		1-2.5 mg/kg q8h or 5-7 mg/kg q24h		1-2.5 mg/kg q8h, or 5-7 mg/kg q24h
Trimethoprim	100 mg q12h or 200 mg q24h		2 mg/kg q12h	
Trimethoprim- sulfamethox- azole (TMP-SMX)	1 tablet[49] q6h or 2 tablets q12h[49]	4-5 mg/kg (TMP) q6-12h	4-5 mg/kg (TMP) q6h	4-5 mg/kg (TMP) q6-12h
Valacyclovir	1 g q8h[51]			

45. When used in combination with other protease inhibitors the ritonavir dose is 100-400 mg PO b.i.d.
46. Soft gelatin capsules.
47. Tetracycline or oxytetracycline. The oral dose of demeclocycline for adults is 600 mg daily in two to four divided doses. The oral dose of minocycline for adults is 100 mg twice a day. The parenteral dose of minocycline is 100-200 mg/day, in one or two doses.
48. Combination formulation: a 3.1-g vial contains 3 g ticarcillin/100 mg clavulanic acid.

USUAL MAXIMUM DOSE/DAY	ADULT DOSAGE IN RENAL FAILURE				
		For Creatinine Clearance (ml/min)			Extra Dose After Hemodialysis
	Dose	80-50	50-10	<10	
1200 mg			Change not required		no
3600 mg			Change not required		
		No change	Not recommended		
80 mg		No change	20 mg q12-24h 15 mg q12-24h	Not recommended	
2 g	0.5-1 g	q24h	q24-72h	q72-96h	yes
8 g	0.5-1 g	q6-8h	q8-12h	q12-24h	yes
300 mg			Not recommended		
2 g			Not recommended		
24-30 g	2-3 g	q4-6h	q6-8h	2 g q12h	yes
18 g		No change[48]	2 g[48] q4-8h	2 g[48] q12h	yes
7 mg/kg	1-1.66 mg/kg	q8-12h	q12-24h	q24-48h	yes
200 mg	100 mg	No change	q18h	q24h	yes
See footnote 50	4-5 mg/kg (TMP)	q12h	q18h	Not recommended	yes
3 g	1 g	q8h	q12-24h	500 mg q24h	

49. Each tablet contains 80 mg trimethoprim and 400 mg sulfamethoxazole. Double-strength tablets are also available; the usual dosage of these is 1 tablet q12h. Suspension contains 40 mg trimethoprim and 200 mg sulfamethoxazole per 5 ml.
50. The usual maximum daily dose is 4 tablets orally or 1200 mg trimethoprim with 6000 mg sulfamethoxazole IV.
51. For herpes zoster. For a first episode of genital herpes, the dosage is 1 g q12h. For recurrence of genital herpes, it is 500 mg q12h. For suppression of genital herpes, it is 1 g q24h.

	ADULTS		CHILDREN	
	ORAL	PARENTERAL	ORAL	PARENTERAL
Valganciclovir	Induction: 900 mg q12h Maintenance: 900 mg q24h		See foot-note 15	
Vancomycin[52]	125-500 mg q6h[53]	1 g IV q12h	12.5 mg/kg q6h[53]	10 mg/kg IV q6h[54,55]
Zalcitabine (ddC)	0.375-0.75 mg q8h		0.005 to 0.01 mg/kg q8h	
Zanamivir	by inhalation 10 mg q12h		>7 years: by inhalation 10 mg q12h	
Zidovudine[9] (AZT)	200 mg q8h or 300 mg q12h		90-180 mg/m^2 q6-8h	

52. Vancomycin should be infused over a period of at least 60 minutes.
53. Only for treatment of pseudomembranous colitis.

USUAL MAXIMUM DOSE/DAY	ADULT DOSAGE IN RENAL FAILURE				
		For Creatinine Clearance (ml/min)			Extra Dose After Hemodialysis
	Dose	80-50	50-10	<10	
1800 mg		Induction: No change	450 mg q12-48h	Not recommended	
		Maintenance: No change	450 mg q24h-2 wks	Not recommended	
2 g	1 g	q12-24h	q24h	See footnote 2	yes
2.25 mg	0.75 mg	No change	q12h	q24h	
20 mg	Change not required				
600 mg		No change	No change	100 mg q6-8h	no*

54. Sixty mg/kg/day may be needed for staphylococcal central-nervous-system infections.
55. Peak serum concentrations should be monitored.

SAFETY OF ANTIMICROBIAL DRUGS IN PREGNANCY

Use of antimicrobial drugs during pregnancy is a frequent cause for concern. The table that follows summarizes the known prenatal risks of most antimicrobials, but the teratogenic potential of many agents remains unknown. The recommendations in the table are based on published data, the opinions of Medical Letter consultants, and on the importance of the drug and the availability of alternatives. Adverse effects not particularly related to pregnancy are not included here; they are summarized in the chapter beginning on page 144. Serum levels of some renally excreted drugs (e.g. β lactams, aminoglycosides) are decreased by 10% to 50% in late pregnancy. For serious infections, maximal recommended doses should be used and serum levels may need to be monitored (OM Korzeniowski, Infect Dis Clin North Am 1995; 9:639).

SOME ANTIMICROBIAL AGENTS IN PREGNANCY

Drug	Toxicity in Pregnancy	Recommendation
Antibacterial		
Amikacin *(Amikin)*	Possible 8th-nerve toxicity in fetus	Caution*
Azithromycin *(Zithromax)*	None known	Probably safe
Aztreonam *(Azactam)*	None known	Probably safe
Cephalosporins[1]	None known	Probably safe

* Use only for strong clinical indication in absence of suitable alternative.

1. Cefaclor (*Ceclor*, others) cefadroxil (*Duricef*, others), cefamandole *(Mandol)*, cefazolin (*Ancef*, others), cefepime *(Maxipime)*, cefdinir *(Omnicef)*, cefditoren *(Spectracef)*, cefixime *(Suprax)*, cefonicid *(Monocid)*, cefoperazone *(Cefobid)*, cefotaxime *(Claforan)*, cefotetan *(Cefotan)*, cefoxitin *(Mefoxin)*, cefpodoxime *(Vantin)*, cefprozil *(Cefzil)*, ceftazidime (*Fortaz*, others), ceftibuten *(Cedax)*, ceftizoxime *(Cefizox)*, ceftriaxone *(Rocephin)*, cefuroxime *(Kefurox, Zinacef)*, cefuroxime axetil *(Ceftin)*, cephalexin (*Keflex*, others), cephapirin (*Cefadyl*, others), cephradine (*Velosef*, others), loracarbef *(Lorabid)*. Experience with newer agents is limited.

Drug	Toxicity in Pregnancy	Recommendation
Chloramphenicol (*Chloromycetin*, others)	Unknown – gray syndrome in newborn	Caution*, especially at term
Cinoxacin (*Cinobac*, others)	Arthropathy in immature animals	Contraindicated
Clarithromycin *(Biaxin)*	Teratogenic in animals	Contraindicated
Clindamycin (*Cleocin*, and others)	None known	Caution*
Dapsone	None known; carcinogenic in rats and mice; hemolytic reactions in neonates	Caution*, especially at term
Dirithromycin *(Dynabac)*	Retarded fetal development in rodents with high doses	Caution*
Ertapenam *(Invanz)*	Decreased total weight in animals	Caution*
Erythromycin estolate (*Ilosone*, and others)	Risk of cholestatic hepatitis appears to be increased in pregnant women	Contraindicated
Erythromycin (*Ery-Tab*, others)	None known	Probably safe but neonatal use has been associated with pyloric stenosis
Fosfomycin *(Monurol)*	Fetal toxicity in rabbits with maternally toxic doses	Caution*
Fluoroquinolones[2]	Arthropathy in immature animals	Caution*
Gentamicin (*Garamycin*, and others)	Possible 8th-nerve toxicity in fetus	Caution*
Imipenem-cilastatin *(Primaxin)*	Toxic in some pregnant animals	Caution*
Kanamycin (*Kantrex*, and others)	Possible 8th-nerve toxicity in fetus	Caution*

* Use only for strong clinical indication in absence of suitable alternative.

2. Ciprofloxacin *(Cipro)*, enoxacin *(Penetrex)*, gatifloxacin *(Tequin)*, levofloxacin *(Levaquin)*, lomefloxacin *(Maxaquin)*, moxifloxacin *(Avelox)*, norfloxacin *(Noroxin)*, ofloxacin *(Floxin)*.

Drug	Toxicity in Pregnancy	Recommendation
Linezolid *(Zyvox)*	Decreased fetal survival in rats	Caution*
Meropenem *(Merrem)*	Unknown	Caution*
Methenamine mandelate (*Mandelamine*, and others)	Unknown	Probably safe
Metronidazole (*Flagyl*, and others)	None known – carcinogenic in rats and mice	Caution*
Nalidixic acid *(NegGram*, and others)	Arthropathy in immature animals; increased intracranial pressure in newborn	Contraindicated
Nitrofurantoin (*Macrodantin*, and others)	Hemolytic anemia in newborn	Caution*; contraindicated at term
Penicillins[3]	None known	Probably safe
Quinupristin/dalfopristin *(Synercid)*	Unknown	Caution*
Spectinomycin *(Trobicin)*	Unknown	Probably safe
Streptomycin	Possible 8th-nerve toxicity in fetus	Caution*
Sulfonamides	Hemolysis in newborn with G-6-PD deficiency; increased risk of kernicterus in newborn; teratogenic in some animal studies	Caution*; contraindicated at term
Tetracyclines[4]	Tooth discoloration and dysplasia, inhibition of bone growth in fetus; hepatic toxicity and azotemia with IV use in pregnant patients with decreased renal function or with overdosage	Contraindicated

* Use only for strong clinical indication in absence of suitable alternative.

3. Amoxicillin (*Amoxil*, and others), amoxicillin/clavulanic acid *(Augmentin)*, ampicillin (*Principen*, and others), ampicillin/sulbactam *(Unasyn)*, carbenicillin indanyl *(Geocillin)*, cloxacillin, dicloxacillin (*Dycill*, and others), nafcillin (*Nafcil*, and others), oxacillin, penicillin G, penicillin V, piperacillin *(Pipracil)*, piperacillin/tazobactam *(Zosyn)*, ticarcillin *(Ticar)*, ticarcillin/clavulanic acid *(Timentin)*. Experience with newer agents is limited.
4. Doxycycline (*Vibramycin*, others), minocycline ((*Minocin*, others), oxytetracycline *(Terramycin)*, demeclocycline *(Declomycin)*, tetracycline hydrochloride (*Sumycin*, others).

Drug	Toxicity in Pregnancy	Recommendation
Tobramycin (*Nebcin*, and others)	Possible 8th-nerve toxicity in fetus	Caution*
Trimethoprim (*Proloprim*, and others)	Folate antagonism; teratogenic in rats	Caution*
Trimethoprim-sulfamethoxazole (*Bactrim*, and others)	Same as sulfonamides and trimethoprim	Caution*; contraindicated at term
Vancomycin (*Vancocin*, and others)	Unknown – possible auditory and renal toxicity in fetus	Caution*
Antifungal		
Amphotericin B (*Fungizone*, and others)	None known	Caution*
Caspofungin *(Cancidas)*	Embryotoxic in animals	Contraindicated
Fluconazole *(Diflucan)*	Teratogenic	Contraindicated for high dose, caution* for single dose
Flucytosine *(Ancobon)*	Teratogenic in rats	Contraindicated
Griseofulvin (*Fulvicin U/F*, and others)	Embryotoxic and teratogenic in animals; carcinogenic in rodents	Contraindicated
Itraconazole *(Sporanox)*	Teratogenic and embryotoxic in rats	Caution*
Ketoconazole *(Nizoral)*	Teratogenic and embryotoxic in rats	Contraindicated
Miconazole *(Monistat i.v.)*	None known	Caution*
Nystatin (*Mycostatin*, and others)	None reported	Probably safe
Antiparasitic		
Albendazole *(Albenza)*	Teratogenic and embryotoxic in animals	Caution*
Atovaquone *(Mepron)*	Maternal and fetal toxicity in animals	Caution*
Atovaquone/proguanil *(Malarone)*	Maternal and fetal toxicity in animals	Caution*
Chloroquine (*Aralen*, and others)	None known with doses recommended for malaria prophylaxis	Probably safe in low doses
Crotamiton *(Eurax)*	Unknown	Caution*
Diloxanide *(Furamide)*	Safety not established	Caution*

* Use only for strong clinical indication in absence of suitable alternative.

Drug	Toxicity in Pregnancy	Recommendation
Furazolidone *(Furoxone)*	None known; carcinogenic in rodents; hemolysis with G-6-PD deficiency in newborn	Caution*; contraindicated at term
Hydroxychloroquine *(Plaquenil)*	None known with doses recommended for malaria prophylaxis	Probably safe in low doses
Iodoquinol (*Yodoxin*, and others)	Unknown	Caution*
Ivermectin *(Stromectol)*	Teratogenic in animals	Contraindicated
Lindane	Absorbed from the skin; potential CNS toxicity in fetus	Contraindicated
Malathion, topical *(Ovide)*	None known	Probably safe
Mebendazole *(Vermox)*	Teratogenic and embryotoxic in rats	Caution*
Mefloquine *(Lariam)*[5]	Teratogenic in animals	Caution*
Metronidazole (*Flagyl*, and others)	None known – carcinogenic in rats and mice	Caution*
Niclosamide *(Niclocide)*	Not absorbed; no known toxicity in fetus	Probably safe
Oxamniquine *(Vansil)*	Embryocidal in animals	Contraindicated
Paromomycin *(Humatin)*	Poorly absorbed; toxicity in fetus unknown	Probably safe
Pentamidine (*Pentam 300, NebuPent*, others)	Safety not established	Caution*
Permethrin (*Nix*, others)	Poorly absorbed; no known toxicity in fetus	Probably safe
Piperazine (*Antepar*, and others)	Unknown	Caution*
Praziquantel *(Biltricide)*	None known	Probably safe
Primaquine	Hemolysis in G-6-PD deficiency	Contraindicated
Pyrantel pamoate (*Antiminth*, others)	Absorbed in small amounts; no known toxicity in fetus	Probably safe
Pyrethrins and piperonyl butoxide (*RID*, others)	Poorly absorbed; no known toxicity in fetus	Probably safe
Pyrimethamine *(Daraprim)*	Teratogenic in animals	Caution*

* Use only for strong clinical indication in absence of suitable alternative.

5. See page 131, footnote 55 and page 135, footnote 72.

Drug	Toxicity in Pregnancy	Recommendation
Pyrimethamine-sulfadoxine *(Fansidar)*	Teratogenic in animals; increased risk of kernicterus in newborn	Caution*, especially at term
Quinacrine *(Atabrine)*	Safety not established	Caution*
Quinine	Large doses can cause abortion; auditory nerve hypoplasia, deafness in fetus; visual changes, limb anomalies, visceral defects also reported	Caution*
Suramin sodium *(Germanin)*	Teratogenic in mice	Caution*
Thiabendazole *(Mintezol)*	None known	Caution*
Antituberculosis		
Capreomycin *(Capastat)*	None known	Caution*
Cycloserine (*Seromycin*, others)	Unknown	Caution*
Ethambutol *(Myambutol)*	None known – teratogenic in animals	Caution*
Ethionamide *(Trecator-SC)*	Teratogenic in animals	Caution*
Isoniazid (*Nydrazid*, others)	Embryocidal in some animals	Probably safe
Pyrazinamide	Unknown	Caution*
Rifabutin *(Mycobutin)*	Unknown	Caution*
Rifampin *(Rifadin, Rimactane)*	Teratogenic in animals	Probably safe
Rifapentine *(Priftin)*	Teratogenic in animals	Caution*
Streptomycin	Possible 8th-nerve toxicity in fetus	Contraindicated
Antiviral		
Abacavir *(Ziagen)*	Teratogenic in animals	Caution*
Acyclovir (*Zovirax*, others)	None known	Caution*
Amantadine (*Symmetrel*, others)	Teratogenic and embryotoxic in rats	Contraindicated
Amprenavir *(Agenerase)*	Teratogenic in animals	Caution*
Cidofovir *(Vistide)*	Embryotoxic in rats and rabbits	Caution*
Delavirdine *(Rescriptor)*	Teratogenic in rats	Caution*
Didanosine (ddI; *Videx)*	None known	Caution*
Efavirenz *(Sustiva)*	Fetal abnormalities in monkeys	Contraindicated

* Use only for strong clinical indication in absence of suitable alternative.

Drug	Toxicity in Pregnancy	Recommendation
Famciclovir *(Famvir)*	Animal toxicity	Contraindicated
Foscarnet *(Foscavir)*	Animal toxicity	Caution*
Ganciclovir *(Cytovene; Vitrasert)*	Teratogenic and embryotoxic in animals	Caution*
Indinavir *(Crixivan)*	None known	Caution*
Interferon alfa (*Intron A*, others)	Large doses cause abortions in animals	Caution*
Pegylated interferon *(PEG-Intron, Pegasys)*	As above	As above
Lamivudine (3TC; *Epivir*)	Unknown	Caution*
Lopinavir/ritonavir *(Kaletra)*	Animal toxicity	Caution*
Nelfinavir *(Viracept)*	No fetal toxicity in animals	Caution*
Nevirapine *(Viramune)*	Decrease in fetal weight in rats	Caution*
Oseltamivir *(Tamiflu)*	Some minor skeletal abnormalities in animals	Caution*
Ribavirin *(Virazole, Rebetol)*	Mutagenic, teratogenic, embryolethal in nearly all species, and possibly carcinogenic in animals	Contraindicated
Rimantadine *(Flumadine)*	Embryotoxic in rats	Contraindicated
Ritonavir *(Norvir)*	Animal toxicity	Caution*
Saquinavir *(Invirase; Fortovase)*	None known	Caution*
Stavudine (d4T; *Zerit*)	Animal toxicity with high doses	Caution*
Tenofovir *(Viread)*	None in animals	Caution*
Valacyclovir *(Valtrex)*	None known	Caution*
Valganciclovir *(Valcyte)*	Teratogenic and embryotoxic in animals	Caution*
Vidarabine *(Vira-A)*	Teratogenic in rats and rabbits	Caution*
Zalcitabine (ddC; *Hivid)*	Teratogenic and embryotoxic in mice	Caution*
Zanamivir *(Relenza)*	None in animals	Caution*
Zidovudine (AZT; *Retrovir)*	Mutagenic *in vitro*	Indicated to prevent HIV infection of fetus

* Use only for strong clinical indication in absence of suitable alternative.

TRADE NAMES

abacavir — *Ziagen* (GlaxoSmithKline)

abacavir-lamivudine-zidovudine — *Trizivir* (GlaxoSmithKline)

Abelcet (Elan) — amphotericin B lipid complex

Actisite (Proctor & Gamble) — tetracycline HCl

* acyclovir — *Zovirax* (GlaxoSmithKline)

Aftate (Schering) — tolnaftate

Agenerase (GlaxoSmithKline) — amprenavir

Ala-Tet (Del-Ray) — tetracycline HCl

alatrofloxacin — *Trovan IV* (Pfizer)

albendazole — *Albenza* (GlaxoSmithKline)

Alferon N (Interferon Sciences) — interferon alfa-n3

* amantadine — *Symmetrel* (Du Pont), others

AmBisome (Fujisawa) — amphotericin B liposomal

amikacin — *Amikin* (Bristol-Myers Squibb)

Amikin (Bristol-Myers Squibb) — amikacin

* aminosalicylic acid — *Paser* (Jacobus)

* amoxicillin — *Amoxil* (GlaxoSmithKline), others

amoxicillin/clavulanic acid — *Augmentin* (GlaxoSmithKline)

Amoxil (GlaxoSmithKline) — amoxicillin

Amphotec (Sequus) — amphotericin B cholesteryl sulfate complex

* amphotericin B — *Fungizone* (Bristol-Myers Squibb), others

amphotericin B cholesteryl sulfate complex — *Amphotec* (Sequus)

amphotericin B lipid complex — *Abelcet* (Elan)

amphotericin B liposomal — *AmBisome* (Fujisawa)

* ampicillin — *Principen* (Bristol-Myers Squibb), others

ampicillin/sulbactam — *Unasyn* (Pfizer)

amprenavir — *Agenerase* (GlaxoSmithKline)

Ancef (GlaxoSmithKline) — cefazolin

Ancobon (Roche) — flucytosine

* *Antiminth* (Pfizer) — pyrantel pamoate

Aralen (Sanofi) — chloroquine

§ *Arsobal* (Aventis, France) — melarsoprol

artemether — *Artenam* (Arenco, Belgium)

atovaquone — *Mepron* (GlaxoSmithKline)

---

* Also available generically.

§ Not commercially available in the US.

atovaquone/proguanil — *Malarone* (GlaxoSmithKline)
Augmentin (GlaxoSmithKline) — amoxicillin/clavulanic acid
Avelox (Bayer) — moxifloxacin
Azactam (Bristol-Myers Squibb) — aztreonam
AZT — see zidovudine
azithromycin — *Zithromax* (Pfizer)
aztreonam — *Azactam* (Bristol-Myers Squibb)

Bactrim (Roche) — trimethoprim-sulfamethoxazole
Beepen-VK (GlaxoSmithKline) — penicillin V
§ benznidazole — *Rochagan* (Roche, Brazil)
Biaxin (Abbott) — clarithromycin
Bicillin LA (Wyeth-Ayerst)— penicillin G benzathine
Biltricide (Bayer) — praziquantel
Bio-cef (Intl Ethic Lab) — cephalexin
§ bithionol — *Bitin* (Tanabe, Japan)
§ *Bitin* — bithionol (Tanabe, Japan)
Brodspec (Truxton) — tetracycline HCl
butoconazole — *Femstat* (Bayer), *Gynazole* (Ther-Rx)

Cancidas (Merck) — caspofungin
Capastat (Dura) — capreomycin
carbenicillin — *Geocillin* (Pfizer)
caspofungin — *Cancidas* (Merck)
Ceclor (Lilly) — cefaclor
cefaclor — *Ceclor* (Lilly)
Cedax (Biovail) — ceftibuten
* cefadroxil — *Duricef* (Bristol-Myers Squibb), others
Cefadyl (Bristol-Myers Squibb) — cephapirin
cefamandole — *Mandol* (Lilly)
* cefazolin — *Ancef* (GlaxoSmithKline), others
cefdinir — *Omnicef* (Abbott)
cefditoren — *Spectracef* (TAP)
cefepime — *Maxipime* (Bristol-Myers Squibb)
cefixime — *Suprax* (Lederle)
Cefizox (Fujisawa) — ceftizoxime
Cefobid (Pfizer) — cefoperazone
cefonicid — *Monocid* (GlaxoSmithKline)
cefoperazone — *Cefobid* (Pfizer)
Cefotan (AstraZeneca) — cefotetan
cefotaxime — *Claforan* (Aventis)
cefotetan — *Cefotan* (Zeneca)
cefoxitin — *Mefoxin* (Merck)
cefpodoxime — *Vantin* (Pharmacia)
cefprozil — *Cefzil* (Bristol-Myers Squibb)
ceftazidime — *Fortaz, Ceptaz, Tazicef* (GlaxoSmithKline), *Tazidime* (Lilly)
ceftibuten — *Cedax* (Biovail)
Ceftin (GlaxoSmithKline) — cefuroxime axetil

* Also available generically.
§ Not commercially available in the US.

ceftizoxime — *Cefizox* (Fujisawa)
ceftriaxone — *Rocephin* (Roche)
cefuroxime — *Kefurox* (Lilly), *Zinacef* (GlaxoSmithKline)
cefuroxime axetil — *Ceftin* (GlaxoSmithKline)
Cefzil (Bristol-Myers Squibb) — cefprozil
* cephalexin — *Keflex* (Dista), others
cephapirin — *Cefadyl* (Bristol-Myers Squibb)
* cephradine — *Velosef* (Bristol-Myers Squibb), others
Ceptaz (GlaxoSmithKline) — ceftazidime
* chloramphenicol — *Chloromycetin* (Parke-Davis), others
Chloromycetin (Parke-Davis) — chloramphenicol
* chloroquine — *Aralen* (Sanofi), others
cidofovir — *Vistide* (Gilead)
Cinobac (Oclassen) — cinoxacin
* cinoxacin — *Cinobac* (Oclassen), others
Cipro (Bayer) — ciprofloxacin
ciprofloxacin — *Cipro* (Bayer)
Claforan (Aventis) — cefotaxime
clarithromycin — *Biaxin* (Abbott)
Cleocin (Pharmacia) — clindamycin
* clindamycin — *Cleocin* (Pharmacia), others
clofazimine — *Lamprene* (Novartis)
clotrimazole — *Mycelex* (Bayer)
* cloxacillin — generic
Cofatrim Fort (Ampharco) — trimethoprim-sulfamethoxazole
colistimethate — *Coly-Mycin* (Parke-Davis)
Coly-Mycin (Parke-Davis) — colistimethate
Combivir (GlaxoSmithKline) — lamivudine-zidovudine
Cotrim (Teva) — trimethoprim-sulfamethoxazole
crotamiton — *Eurax* (Westwood-Squibb)
Crixivan (Merck) — indinavir
§ *Cryptaz* (Romark) — nitazoxanide
* cycloserine — *Seromycin* (Dura), others
Cytovene (Roche) — ganciclovir

ddC — see didanosine
ddI — see zalcitabine
* dapsone — generic (Jacobus)
Daraprim (GlaxoSmithKline) — pyrimethamine
Declomycin (Lederle) — demeclocycline
delavirdine — *Rescriptor* (Pharmacia)
demeclocycline — *Declomycin* (Lederle)
Denavir (Novartis) — penciclovir
* dicloxacillin — *Dycill* (GlaxoSmithKline), others
didanosine — *Videx* (Bristol-Myers Squibb)
diethylcarbamazine — *Hetrazan* (Lederle)
Diflucan (Pfizer) — fluconazole

* Also available generically.
§ Not commercially available in the US.

§ diloxanide furoate — *Furamide* (Knoll, U.K.)
dirithromycin — *Dynabac* (Muro)
Doryx (Warner Chilcott) — doxycycline
* doxycycline — *Vibramycin* (Pfizer), others
Duricef (Bristol-Myers Squibb) — cefadroxil
Dycill (GlaxoSmithKline) — dicloxacillin
Dynabac (Muro) — dirithromycin
Dynapen (Bristol-Myers Squibb) — dicloxacillin
* erythromycin — *Erythrocin* (Abbott), others
* erythromycin-sulfisoxazole — *Pediazole* (Ross/Abbott), others
Eryzole (Alra) — erythromycin-sulfisoxazole
ethambutol — *Myambutol* (Lederle)
ethionamide — *Trecator-SC* (Wyeth-Ayerst)
Eurax (Westwood-Squibb) — crotamiton
Exelderm (Westwood-Squibb) — sulconazole

E.E.S. (Abbott) — erythromycin
efavirenz — *Sustiva* (DuPont)
§ *Egaten* (Novartis) — triclabendazole
§ eflornithine — *Ornidyl* (Aventis)
Elimite (Allergan) — permethrin
Emtet-500 (EconoMed) — tetracycline HCl
E-Mycin (Knoll) — erythromycin
enoxacin — *Penetrex* (Aventis)
Epivir (GlaxoSmithKline) — lamivudine
ertapenem — *Invanz* (Merck)
Ery-Tab (Abbott) — erythromycin
ERYC (Parke-Davis) — erythromycin
Erythrocin (Abbott) — erythromycin

famciclovir — *Famvir* (GlaxoSmithKline)
Famvir (GlaxoSmithKline) — famciclovir
Fansidar (Roche) — pyrimethamine-sulfadoxine
§ *Fasigyn* (Pfizer) — tinidazole
Femstat (Bayer) — butoconazole
Flagyl (Searle) — metronidazole
Floxin (Ortho-McNeil) — ofloxacin
fluconazole — *Diflucan* (Pfizer)
flucytosine — *Ancobon* (Roche)
Flumadine (Forest) — rimantadine
fomivirsen — *Vitravene* (Novartis)
Fortaz (GlaxoSmithKline) — ceftazidime
Fortovase (Roche) — saquinavir
foscarnet — *Foscavir* (AstraZeneca)

* Also available generically.
§ Not commercially available in the US.

Foscavir (AstraZeneca) — foscarnet
fosfomycin — *Monurol* (Forest)
Fulvicin P/G (Schering) — griseofulvin
Fulvicin U/F (Schering) — griseofulvin
Fungizone (Bristol-Myers Squibb) — amphotericin B
Furacin (Roberts) — nitrofurazone
Furadantin (Dura) — nitrofurantoin
§ *Furamide* (Knoll, U.K.) — diloxanide furoate
furazolidone — *Furoxone* (Roberts)
Furoxone (Roberts) — furazolidone

ganciclovir — *Cytovene* (Roche); *Vitrasert* (Bauch & Lomb)
Gantrisin (Roche) — sulfisoxazole
Garamycin (Schering) — gentamicin
gatifloxacin — *Tequin* (Bristol-Myers Squibb)
* gentamicin — *Garamycin* (Schering), others
Geocillin (Pfizer) — carbenicillin
§ *Glucantime* (Aventis, France) — meglumine antimoniate
G-Mycin (Bolan) — gentamicin
Grifulvin V (Ortho) — griseofulvin
Grisactin (Wyeth-Ayerst) — griseofulvin
* griseofulvin — *Fulvicin U/F* (Schering), others
Gris-PEG (Allergan) — griseofulvin
Gynazole (Ther-Rx) — butoconazole

§ *Halfan* (GlaxoSmithKline) — halofantrine
§ halofantrine — *Halfan* (GlaxoSmithKline)
Hetrazan (Lederle) — diethylcarbamazine
Hiprex (Aventis) — methenamine hippurate
Hivid (Roche) — zalcitabine
Humatin (Parke-Davis) — paromomycin
hydroxychloroquine — *Plaquenil* (Sanofi-Synthelabo)

Ilosone (Dista) — erythromycin estolate
imipenem-cilastatin — *Primaxin* (Merck)
indinavir — *Crixivan* (Merck)
Infanz (Merck) — ertapenem
Infergen (Amgen) — interferon alfacon-1
interferon alfa-2a — *Roferon-A* (Roche)
interferon alfa-2a, pegylated — *Pegasys* (Roche)
interferon alfa-2b — *Intron A* (Schering)
interferon alfa-2b, pegylated — *PEG-Intron* (Schering)
interferon alfa-n3 — *Alferon N* (Interferon Sciences)

* Also available generically.
§ Not commercially available in the US.

interferon alfacon-1 — *Infergen* (Amgen)
Intron A (Schering) — interferon alfa-2b
Invirase (Roche) — saquinavir
* iodoquinol — *Yodoxin* (Glenwood), others
* isoniazid — *Nydrazid* (Bristol-Myers Squibb)
itraconazole — *Sporanox* (Janssen)
ivermectin — *Stromectol* (Merck)

Kaletra (Abbott) — lopinavir/ritonavir
* kanamycin — *Kantrex* (Bristol-Myers Squibb), others
Kantrex (Bristol-Myers Squibb) — kanamycin
Keflex (Dista) — cephalexin
Keftab (Dista) — cephalexin
Kefurox (Lilly) — cefuroxime
Kefzol (Lilly) — cefazolin
ketoconazole — *Nizoral* (Janssen)

lamivudine — *Epivir* (GlaxoSmithKline)
lamivudine-zidovudine — *Combivir* (GlaxoSmithKline)
lamivudine-zidovudine-abacavir — *Trizivir* (GlaxoSmithKline)
§ *Lampit* (Bayer, Germany) — nifurtimox
Lamprene (Novartis) — clofazimine
Lariam (Roche) — mefloquine
Ledercillin VK (Lederle) — penicillin V
levofloxacin — *Levaquin* (Ortho-McNeil)
Lincocin (Pharmacia) — lincomycin
* lincomycin — *Lincocin* (Pharmacia)
Lincorex (Hyrex) — lincomycin
linezolid — *Zyvox* (Pharmacia)
lomefloxacin — *Maxaquin* (Searle)
lopinavir/ritonavir — *Kaletra* (Abbott)
Lorabid (Lilly) — loracarbef
loracarbef — *Lorabid* (Lilly)
Lyphocin (Lypho-Med) — vancomycin

Macrobid (Proctor & Gamble) — nitrofurantoin
Macrodantin (Proctor & Gamble) — nitrofurantoin
Malarone (GlaxoSmithKline) — atovaquone/proguanil
malathion — *Ovide* (Medicis)
Mandelamine (Warner Chilcott) — methenamine mandelate
Mandol (Lilly) — cefamandole
Marcillin (Marnel) — ampicillin
Maxaquin (Searle) — lomefloxacin
Maxipime (Bristol-Myers Squibb) — cefepime
mebendazole — *Vermox* (Janssen)
mefloquine — *Lariam* (Roche)
Mefoxin (Merck) — cefoxitin

---

* Also available generically.
§ Not commercially available in the US.

§ meglumine antimoniate — *Glucantime* (Aventis, France)
§ melarsoprol — *Arsobal* (Aventis, France)
meropenem — *Merrem* (AstraZeneca)
Merrem (AstraZeneca) — meropenem
methenamine hippurate — *Hiprex* (Aventis), *Urex* (3M)
* methenamine mandelate — *Mandelamine* (Warner Chilcott), others
* metronidazole — *Flagyl* (Searle), others
* miconazole — *Monistat* (Ortho-McNeil), others
Minocin (Lederle) — minocycline
* minocycline — *Minocin* (Lederle), others
Mintezol (Merck) — thiabendazole
Monistat (Ortho-McNeil) — miconazole
Monodox (Oclassen) — doxycycline
Monurol (Forest) — fosfomycin
moxifloxacin — *Avelox* (Bayer)
Myambutol (Lederle) — ethambutol
Mycelex (Bayer) — clotrimazole
Mycobutin (Pharmacia) — rifabutin
Mycostatin (Bristol-Myers Squibb) — nystatin
My-E (Seneca) — erythromycin

nafcillin — *Unipen* (Wyeth-Ayerst)
* nalidixic acid — *NegGram* (Sanofi), others
Nallpen (Baxter) — nafcillin
Natacyn (Alcon) — natamycin
natamycin — *Natacyn* (Alcon)
Nebcin (Lilly) — tobramycin
NebuPent (Fujisawa) — pentamidine
NegGram (Sanofi) — nalidixic acid
nelfinavir — *Viracept* (Pfizer)
* neomycin — many manufacturers
Neutrexin (US Bioscience) — trimetrexate
nevirapine — *Viramune* (Boehringer Ingelheim)
§ niclosamide — *Yomesan* (Bayer, Germany)
§ nifurtimox — *Lampit* (Bayer, Germany)
Nilstat (Lederle) — nystatin
§ nitazoxanide — *Cryptaz* (Romark)
* nitrofurantoin — *Macrodantin* (Proctor & Gamble), others
* nitrofurazone — *Furacin* (Roberts), others
Nix (GlaxoSmithKline) — permethrin
Nizoral (Janssen) — ketoconazole
norfloxacin — *Noroxin* (Merck)
Noroxin (Merck) — norfloxacin
Norvir (Abbott) — ritonavir
Nydrazid (Bristol-Myers Squibb) — isoniazid
* nystatin — *Mycostatin* (Bristol-Myers Squibb), others
Nystex (Savage) — nystatin

---

* Also available generically.
§ Not commercially available in the US.

ofloxacin — *Floxin* (Ortho-McNeil)
Omnicef (Abbott) — cefdinir
Omnipen (Wyeth-Ayerst) — ampicillin
§ ornidazole — *Tiberal* (Hoffmann LaRoche, Switzerland)
§ *Ornidyl* (Aventis) — eflornithine
oseltamivir — *Tamiflu* (Roche/Gilead)
Ovide (Medicis) — malathion
* oxacillin — generic
oxamniquine — *Vansil* (Pfizer)
oxytetracycline — *Terramycin* (Pfizer)

§ *Paludrine* (Ayerst, Canada, ICI, U.K.) — proguanil
Panmycin (Pharmacia) — tetracycline HCl
paromomycin — *Humatin* (Parke-Davis)
Paser (Jacobus) — aminosalicylic acid
Pediazole (Ross/Abbott) — erythromycin-sulfisoxazole
§ *Pegasys* (Roche) — pegylated interferon alfa 2a
PEG-Intron (Schering) — pegylated interferon alfa 2b
penciclovir — *Denavir* (Novartis)
Penetrex (Aventis) — enoxacin
* penicillin G — many manufacturers
penicillin G benzathine — *Bicillin LA* (Wyeth-Ayerst), *Permapen* (Pfizer)
* penicillin G procaine — many manufacturers
* penicillin V — many manufacturers
Pentam 300 (Fujisawa) — pentamidine
* pentamidine isethionate — *Pentam 300* (Fujisawa), *NebuPent* (Fujisawa), others
§ *Pentostam* (GlaxoSmithKline, U.K.) — sodium stibogluconate
Pen-V (Zenith Goldline) — penicillin V
Permapen (Pfizer) — penicillin G benzathine
* permethrin — *Elimite* (Allergan), *Nix* (GlaxoSmithKline)
piperacillin — *Pipracil* (Lederle)
piperacillin/tazobactam — *Zosyn* (Lederle)
Pipracil (Lederle) — piperacillin
Plaquenil (Sanofi- Synthelabo) — hydroxychloroquine
* polymyxin B — generic
praziquantel — *Biltricide* (Bayer)
Priftin (Aventis) — rifapentine
primaquine phosphate (Sanofi) — generic
Primaxin (Merck) — imipenem-cilastatin sodium
Principen (Bristol-Myers Squibb) — ampicillin
§ proguanil — *Paludrine* (Ayerst, Canada; ICI, U.K.)
proguanil/atovaquone — *Malarone* (GlaxoSmithKline)
Proloprim (GlaxoSmithKline) — trimethoprim
Pronto (Del) — pyrethrins with piperonyl butoxide

* Also available generically.
§ Not commercially available in the US.

Protostat (Ortho-McNeil) — metronidazole
* pyrantel pamoate — *Antiminth* (Pfizer), others
* pyrazinamide — generic
* pyrethrins with piperonyl butoxide — *RID* (Pfizer), others

pyrimethamine — *Daraprim* (GlaxoSmithKline)

pyrimethamine-sulfadoxine — *Fansidar* (Roche)

* quinidine gluconate — many manufacturers

§ quinine dihydrochloride
* quinine sulfate — many manufacturers

quinupristin–dalfopristin — *Synercid* (Aventis)

Rebetol (Schering) — ribavirin

Rebetron (Schering) — ribavirin-interferon alfa-2b

Relenza (GlaxoSmithKline) — zanamivir

Rescriptor (Pharmacia) — delavirdine

Retrovir (GlaxoSmithKline) — zidovudine

ribavirin — *Virazole* (ICN); *Rebetol* (Schering)

ribavirin-interferon alfa-2b *Rebetron* (Schering)

RID (Pfizer) — pyrethrins with piperonyl butoxide

rifabutin — *Mycobutin* (Pharmacia)

Rifadin (Aventis) — rifampin

Rifamate (Aventis) — rifampin-isoniazid

rifampin — *Rimactane* (Novartis), *Rifadin* (Aventis)

rifampin-isoniazid — *Rifamate* (Aventis)

rifapentine — *Priftin* (Aventis)

Rifater (Aventis) — rifampin, isoniazid and pyrazinamide

Rimactane (Novartis) — rifampin

rimantadine — *Flumadine* (Forest)

ritonavir — *Norvir* (Abbott)

ritonavir/lopinavir — *Kaletra* (Abbott)

Rocephin (Roche) — ceftriaxone

§ *Rochagan* (Roche, Brazil) — benznidazole

Roferon-A (Roche) — interferon alfa-2a

§ *Rovamycine* (Aventis) — spiramycin

saquinavir — *Fortovase; Invirase* (Roche)

Septra (GlaxoSmithKline) — trimethoprim-sulfamethoxazole

Seromycin (Lilly) — cycloserine

§ sodium stibogluconate — *Pentostam* (GlaxoSmithKline, U.K.)

Soxa (Vita Elixir) — sulfisoxazole

spectinomycin — *Trobicin* (Pharmacia)

Spectracef (TAP) — cefditoren

§ spiramycin — *Rovamycine* (Aventis)

Sporanox (Janssen) — itraconazole

---

* Also available generically.

§ Not commercially available in the US.

stavudine — *Zerit* (Bristol-Myers Squibb)
* streptomycin — generic
Stromectol (Merck) — ivermectin
sulconazole — *Exelderm* (Westwood-Squibb)
Sulfatrim — trimethoprim-sulfamethoxazole
* sulfisoxazole — *Gantrisin* (Roche), others
Sumycin (Bristol-Myers Squibb) — tetracycline HCl
Suprax (Lederle) — cefixime
§ suramin — (Bayer, Germany)
Suspen (Circle) — penicillin V
Sustiva (DuPont) — efavirenz
Symmetrel (Du Pont) — amantadine
Synercid (Aventis) — quinupristin-dalfopristin

Tamiflu (Roche/Gilead) — oseltamivir
TAO (Pfizer) — troleandomycin
Tazicef (GlaxoSmithKline) — ceftazidime
Tazidime (Lilly) — ceftazidime
Tequin (Bristol-Myers Squibb) — gatifloxacin
Terramycin (Pfizer) — oxytetracycline
Tetracap (Circle) — tetracycline HCl
Tetracon (Consolidated Midland) — tetracycline HCl
* tetracycline HCl — *Sumycin* (Bristol-Myers Squibb), others
thiabendazole — *Mintezol* (Merck)
§ *Tiberal* (Hoffmann LaRoche, Switzerland) — ornidazole
Ticar (GlaxoSmithKline) — ticarcillin
ticarcillin — *Ticar* (GlaxoSmithKline)
ticarcillin/clavulanic acid — *Timentin* (GlaxoSmithKline)
Timentin (GlaxoSmithKline) — ticarcillin/clavulanic acid
§ tinidazole — *Fasigyn* (Pfizer)
tioconazole — *Vagistat* (Bristol-Myers Squibb)
* tobramycin — *Nebcin* (Lilly), others
* tolnaftate — *Aftate* (Schering), others
Trecator-SC (Wyeth-Ayerst) — ethionamide
§ triclabendazole — *Egaten* (Novartis)
trifluridine — *Viroptic* (GlaxoSmithKline)
* trimethoprim — *Proloprim* (GlaxoSmithKline), others
* trimethoprim-sulfamethoxazole — *Bactrim* (Roche), *Septra* (GlaxoSmithKline), others
trimetrexate — *Neutrexin* (US Bioscience)
Trimox (Bristol-Myers Squibb) — amoxicillin
Trimpex (Roche) — trimethoprim
* trisulfapyrimidines — Triple Sulfa (Allscripts), others
Trizivir (GlaxoSmithKline) — abacavir, lamivudine, zidovudine

* Also available generically.
§ Not commercially available in the US.

Trobicin (Pharmacia) — spectinomycin
troleandomycin — *TAO* (Pfizer)
trovafloxacin — *Trovan* (Pfizer)
Trovan (Pfizer) — trovafloxacin
Truxazole (Truxton) — sulfisoxazole
Truxcillin VK (Truxton) — penicillin V

Unasyn (Pfizer) — ampicillin/sulbactam
Unipen (Wyeth-Ayerst) — nafcillin
Urex (Virco) — methenamine hippurate

Vagistat (Bristol-Myers Squibb) — tioconazole
valacyclovir — *Valtrex* (GlaxoSmithKline)
valganciclovir — *Valcyte* (Roche)
Valcyte (Roche) — valganciclovir
Valtrex (GlaxoSmithKline) — valacyclovir
Vancocin (Lilly) — vancomycin
Vancoled (Lederle) — vancomycin
* vancomycin — *Vancocin* (Lilly), others
Vansil (Pfizer) — oxamniquine
Vantin (Pharmacia) — cefpodoxime
V-cillin K (Lilly) — penicillin
Veetids (Bristol-Myers Squibb) — penicillin V
Velosef (Bristol-Myers Squibb) — cephradine
Vermox (Janssen) — mebendazole
Vibramycin (Pfizer) — doxycycline
Vibra-Tabs (Pfizer) — doxycycline
vidarabine — *Vira-A* (Parke-Davis)
Videx (Bristol-Myers Squibb) — didanosine
Vira-A (Parke-Davis) — vidarabine
Viracept (Pfizer) — nelfinavir
Viramune (Boehringer Ingelheim) — nevirapine
Virazole (ICN) — ribavirin
Viread (Gilead) — tenofovir
Viroptic (GlaxoSmithKline) — trifluridine
Vistide (Gilead) — cidofovir
Vitrasert (Bausch & Lomb) — ganciclovir
Vitravene (Novartis) — fomivirsen

Wesmycin (Wesley) — tetracycline HCl
Wycillin (Wyeth-Ayerst) — penicillin G
Wymox (Wyeth-Ayerst) — amoxicillin

Yodoxin (Glenwood) — iodoquinol
§ *Yomesan* (Bayer, Germany) — niclosamide

zalcitabine — *Hivid* (Roche)
zanamivir — *Relenza* (GlaxoSmithKline)

* Also available generically.
§ Not commercially available in the US.

Zerit (Bristol-Myers Squibb) — stavudine
Ziagen (GlaxoSmithKline) — abacavir
zidovudine — *Retrovir* (GlaxoSmithKline)
zidovudine-lamivudine — *Combivir* (GlaxoSmithKline)
zidovudine-lamivudine-abacavir — *Trizivir* (GlaxoSmithKline)
Zinacef (GlaxoSmithKline) — cefuroxime
Zithromax (Pfizer) — azithromycin
Zosyn (Lederle) — piperacillin/tazobactam
Zovirax (GlaxoSmithKline) — acyclovir
Zyvox (Pharmacia) — linezolid

---

* Also available generically.
§ Not commercially available in the US.

INDEX

Note: Page numbers in bold type indicate major references.

Abacavir, **90**
  adverse effects, 144
  dosage, 162
  in pregnancy, 187
Acanthamoeba, 120
Acanthamoeba keratitis, 120
Acid fast bacilli, 50
Acinetobacter, 47
Actinomyces israelii, 50
Actinomycosis, 50
Acyclovir, **74**
  adverse effects, 144
  dosage, 85, 86, 87, 106, 162
  in pregnancy, 187
  indications, 109
Aeromonas, 47
Albendazole
  adverse effects, 144
  in pregnancy, 185
  indications and dosage, 121, 122, 123, 124, 125, 127, 128, 136, 139, 140, 141, 142
Amantadine, **75**
  adverse effects, 144
  dosage, 86, 162
  in pregnancy, 187
Amebiasis, 120
Amebic meningoencephalitis, primary, 121
Amikacin, 5
  adverse, effects, 69, 145
  dosage, 73, 162
  in pregnancy, 182
  indications, 67
Aminoglycosides, 5
  indications, 101
Aminosalicylic acid, 6
  adverse effects, 70, 145
  dosage, 73
  indications, 67
Amoxicillin, 6
  adverse effects, 154
  dosage, 64, 65, 103, 162
  in pregnancy, 184
  indications, 100
Amoxicillin-clavulanic acid, 6
  adverse effects, 154
  dosage, 162
  in pregnancy, 184
  indications, 63
Amphotericin B, **114**,
  adverse effects, 145
  dosage, 111, 112, 113, 162
  in pregnancy, 185
  indications, 121, 128
  lipid formulations, 114
Ampicillin, 7
  adverse effects, 154
  dosage, 64, 65, 162
  in pregnancy, 184
Ampicillin-sulbactam, 7
  adverse effects, 154
  dosage, 104, 162
  in pregnancy, 184
  indications, 63
Amprenavir, **94**
  adverse effects, 145
  dosage, 164
  in pregnancy, 187
  indications, 68
Ancylostoma caninum, 121
Ancylostoma duodenale, 128
Angiostrongyliasis, 122
Angiostrongylus cantonensis, 122
Angiostrongylus costaricensis, 122
Anisakiasis, 122
Anisakis, 122
Anthrax, 43
Artemether
  adverse effects, 145
  indications and dosage, 131, 133
Artesunate
  adverse effects, 145
  indications and dosage, 131

Ascariasis, 122
Ascaris lumbricoides, 122
Aspergillosis, 111
Atovaquone
  adverse effects, 145
  in pregnancy, 185
  indications and dosage, 122, 130, 134, 135, 137, 138, 140
Atovaquone/proguanil
  in pregnancy, 185
  indications and dosage, 130, 134, 135
Azithromycin, 14
  adverse effects, 145
  dosage, 64, 103, 106, 164
  in pregnacy, 182
  indications, 99, 100, 108, 121, 122
AZT, **88**
Aztreonam, 7
  adverse effects, 146
  dosage, 164
  in pregnancy, 182

Babesia, 122
Babesiosis, 122
Bacillary angiomatosis, 47
Bacillus anthracis, 43
Bacillus cereus subtilis, 43
Bacitracin, 7
  adverse effects, 146
  indications and dosage, 127
Bacterial vaginosis, 48
Bacteroides, 44
Balamuthia mandrillaria, 121
Balantidiasis, 123
Balantidium coli, 123
Balnei, 50
Bartonella, 47
Baylisascariasis, 123
Baylisascaris procyonis, 123
Benznidazole
  adverse effects, 146
  indications and dosage, 141
Bilharziasis, 138
Bite wounds, 63
Bithionol
  adverse effects, 146
  indications and dosage, 126
Blastocystis hominis, 123
Blastomycosis, 111
Bordetella pertussis, 47
Borrelia burgdorferi, 52
Borrelia recurrentis, 52
Brachiola vesicularum, 136
Branhamella, 43
Brucella, 48
Brugia malayi, 125
Brugia timori, 125
Burkholderia cepacia, 48
Burkholeria mallei, 48
Burkholeria pseudomallei, 48
Butoconazole, indications, 102

Calymmatobacterium granulomatis, 48
Campylobacter fetus, 44
Campylobacter jejuni, 44
Candidiasis, 112
  vulvovaginal, **102**, **105**
Capillaria philippinensis, 123
Capillariasis, 123
Capnocytophaga canimorsus, 48
Capreomycin, 7
  adverse effects, 69, 146
  dosage, 73
  in pregnancy, 187
  indications, 67
Carbapenems, 7
Carbenicillin, 8
  adverse effects, 154
  dosage, 164
  in pregnancy, 184
Caspofungin, **115**
  dosage, 111, 112, 164
  in pregnancy, 185
Cat scratch bacillus, 47
Cefaclor, 10
  adverse effects, 146
  dosage, 164
  in pregnancy, 182

Cefadroxil, 10
adverse effects, 146
dosage, 64, 164
in pregnancy, 182
Cefamandole, 9
adverse effects, 146
dosage, 164
in pregnancy, 182
Cefazolin, 8
adverse effects, 146
dosage, 61, 62, 63, 64, 164
in pregnancy, 182
indications, 55
Cefdinir, 10
adverse effects, 146
dosage, 164
in pregnancy, 182
Cefditoren, 10
adverse effects, 146
dosage, 164
in pregnancy, 182
Cefepime, 9
adverse effects, 146
dosage, 164
in pregnancy, 182
Cefixime, 10
adverse effects, 146
dosage, 105, 164
in pregnancy, 182
indications, 100
Cefonicid, 9
adverse effects, 146
dosage, 164
in pregnancy, 182
Cefoperazone, 9
adverse effects, 146
dosage, 164
in pregnancy, 182
Cefotaxime, 9
adverse effects, 146
dosage, 166
in pregnancy, 182
Cefotetan, 9
adverse effects, 146
dosage, 61, 62, 104, 164
in pregnancy, 182
indications, 55, 101
Cefoxitin, 9
adverse effects, 146
dosage, 61, 62, 166
in pregnancy, 182
indications, 55, 101
Cefpodoxime, 10
adverse effect, 146
dosage 166
in pregnancy, 182
Cefprozil, 10
adverse effects, 146
dosage, 166
in pregnancy, 182
Ceftazidime, 9
adverse effects, 146
dosage, 166
in pregnancy, 182
Ceftibuten, 10
adverse effect, 146
dosage, 166
in pregnancy, 182
Ceftizoxime, 9
adverse effects, 146
dosage, 166
in pregnancy, 182
Ceftriaxone, 9
adverse effects, 146
dosage, 103, 104, 105, 166
in pregnancy, 182
indications, 100, 108
Cefuroxime, 9
adverse effects, 146
dosage, 61, 63, 166
in pregnancy, 182
Cefuroxime axetil, 10
adverse effects, 146
dosage, 166
in pregnancy, 182
Cephalexin, 10
adverse effects, 146
dosage, 64, 166
in pregnancy, 182
Cephalosporins, 8
adverse effects, 146
in pregnancy, 182

Cephapirin, 8
adverse effects, 146
dosage, 166
in pregnancy, 182
Cephradine, 10
adverse effects, 146
dosage, 166
Cervicitis, 99
Chagas' disease, 141
Chancroid, 48, **106**, **108**
Chinese liver fluke, 126
Chlamydia pneumoniae, 51
Chlamydia psittaci, 51
Chlamydia trachomatis, 51, **99**, **103**
Chloramphenicol, 10
adverse effects, 146
dosage, 166
in pregnancy, 183
Chlorhexidine, 120, 121
Chloroquine
adverse effects, 147
in pregnancy, 185
indications and dosage, 132, 133, 134, 135
Cholera, 50
Cidofovir, **76**
adverse effects, 147
dosage, 84, 166
in pregnancy, 187
Cilastatin, 8
Cinoxacin, 18
adverse effects, 147
dosage, 168
in pregnancy, 183
Ciprofloxacin, 12
adverse effects, 149
dosage, 62, 73, 106, 168
in pregnancy, 183
indications, 100, 108, 124, 128
Clarithromycin, 15
adverse effects, 147
dosage, 64, 168
in pregnancy, 183
indications, 121
Clavulanic acid, 6, 20
Clindamycin, 11
adverse effects, 147
dosage, 62, 63, 64, 104, 105, 168
in pregnancy, 183
indications, 101, 122, 130, 138, 140
Clofazimine, 11
adverse effects, 147
Clonorchis sinensis, 126
Clostridium difficile, 43
Clostridium perfringens, 43
Clostridium tetani, 43
Clotrimazole
dosage, 111
indications, 102
Cloxacillin, 17
adverse effects, 154
dosage, 168
in pregnancy, 184
CMV, 76, 77, 78, 84
Coccidioidomycosis, 112
Colistimethate, 18
adverse effects, 155
Colistin sulfate, 18
Corynebacterium diphtheriae, 44
Corynebacterium JK group, 44
Cost
of drugs for HIV, **96**
of oral antibacterials, **53**
of viral drugs, **84**
Creeping eruption, 123
Crotamiton, 138
adverse effects, 147
in pregnancy, 185
Cryptococcosis, 112
Cryptosporidiosis, 123
Cryptosporidium, 123
Cutaneous larva migrans, 123
Cycloserine, 11
adverse effects, 147
dosage, 73, 168
in pregnancy, 187
indications, 67
Cyclospora, 124
Cysticercosis, 139
Cysticercus cellulosae, 139
Cytomegalovirus, 76, 77, 78, 84

Dalfopristin, 18
Dapsone
  adverse effects, 147
  in pregnancy, 183
  indications, 137, 140
DDC, **90**
DDI, **89**
Delavirdine, **92**
  adverse effects, 148
  dosage, 168
  in pregnancy, 187
Demeclocycline, 20
  adverse effects, 157
  dosage, 178
  in pregnancy, 184
Dicloxacillin, 17
  adverse effects, 154
  dosage, 168
  in pregnancy, 184
Didanosine, **89**
  adverse effects, 148
  dosage, 168
  in pregnancy, 188
Dientamoeba fragilis, 124
Diethylcarbamazine
  adverse effects, 150
  indications and dosage, 125, 126
Diloxanide furoate
  adverse effects, 148
  in pregnancy, 186
  indications and dosage, 120
Diphtheria, 44
Diphyllobothrium latum, 139
Dipylidium caninum, 139
Dirithromycin, 15
  adverse effects, 148
  dosage, 168
  in pregnancy, 183
Disk diffusion tests, **27**
Dosage
  antimicrobials agents, **160**
  endocarditis prophylaxis, **64**
  fungal infections, **111**
  HIV, **96**
  parasitic infections, **120**
  sexually transmitted diseases, **103**
  surgical prophylaxis, **61**
  tuberculosis, **72**
  viral infections, **84**
Doxycycline, 20
  adverse effects, 157
  dosage, 62, 103, 104, 105, 168
  in pregnancy, 184
  indications, 99, 101, 125, 130, 131, 134, 135
Dracunculus medinensis, 124

Echinococcus granulosus, 139
Echinococcus multilocularis, 139
Efavirenz, **91**
  adverse effects, 148
  dosage, 168
  in pregnancy, 188
  indications, 68
Eflornithine
  adverse effects, 148
  indications and dosage, 141, 142
Ehrlichia chaffeensis, 51
Ehrlichia ewingii, 51
Ehrlichia phagocytophilia, 51
Ehrlichiosis, 51
Eikenella corrodens, 48
Encephalitozoon hellem, 136
Encephalitozoon intestinalis, 136
Encephlitozoon cuniculi, 136
Endocarditis, 40
  prophylaxis, **64**
Enoxacin, 12
  adverse effects, 149
  dosage, 168
  in pregnancy, 183
Entamoeba histolytica, 120
Entamoeba polecki, 124
Enterobacter, 44
Enterobius vermicularis, 124
Enterococcus, 40
Enterocytozoon bieneusi, 136
Eosinophilic enterocolitis, 121
Epididymitis, **100, 103**
Ertapenem, 7
  dosage, 168
  in pregnancy, 183

Erysipelothrix rhusiopathiae, 44
Erythromycin, 15
  adverse effects, 148
  dosage, 61, 103, 106, 168
  in pregnancy, 183
  indications, 99, 100, 108
Erythromycin-sulfisoxazole, 15, 19
Escherichia coli, 45
Ethambutol, 12
  adverse effects, 70, 148
  dosage, 72, 170
  in pregnancy, 187
  indications, 66
Ethionamide, 12
  adverse effects, 149
  dosage, 73, 170
  indications, 67
  pregnancy, 187

Famciclovir, **77**
  adverse effects, 149
  dosage, 85, 86, 87, 106, 170
  in pregnancy, 188
  indications, 109
Fasciola hepatica, 126
Fasciolopsis buski, 126
Filariasis, 125
Fluconazole, **116**
  adverse effects, 149
  dosage, 105, 111, 112, 113, 170
  in pregnancy, 185
  indications, 102, 121
Flucytosine, **115**
  adverse effects, 149
  dosage, 112, 170
  in pregnancy, 185
  indications, 121
Fluke infection, 126
Fluoroquinolones, 12
  adverse effects, 70, 149
  in pregnancy, 183
Folinic acid, 138, 140
Fomivirsen, **77**
  dosage, 84
Foscarnet, **77**
  adverse effects, 149
  dosage, 84, 86, 87, 170
  in pregnancy, 188
Fosfomycin, 13
  adverse effects, 149
  dosage, 170
  in pregnancy, 183
Francisella tularensis, 48
Fumagillin, 136
Fungal infections, drugs for, **111**
Furazolidone, 13
  adverse effects, 149
  in pregnancy, 186
  indications and dosage, 127
Fusariosis, 113
Fusobacterium, 48

Ganciclovir, **78**
  adverse effects, 150
  dosage, 84, 170
  in pregnancy, 188
Gardnerella vaginalis, 48, 102
Gatifloxacin, 13
  adverse effects, 149
  dosage, 73, 170
  in pregnancy, 183
G-CSF, 79
Gentamicin, 5
  adverse effects, 150
  dosage, 62, 63, 65, 104, 170
  in pregnancy, 183
Giardiasis, 127
Glanders, 48
GM-CSF, 79
Gnathostoma spinigerum, 127
Gnathostomiasis, 127
Gongylonema, 127
Gongylonemiasis, 127
Gonococcus, 43
Gonorrhea, **100**, **104**
Granulocyte-colony-stimulating factor, 79
Granuloma inguinale, 48
Griseofulvin
  adverse effects, 150

dosage, 170
in pregnancy, 185
Guinea worm infection, 124

Haemophilus ducreyi, 48, 108
Haemophilus influenzae, 49
Halofantrine
adverse effects, 150
indications and dosage, 131, 132
Hantavirus, 82
Haverhill fever, 49
Helicobacter pylori, 45
Hemorrhagic fever, 82
Hepatitis B, 79, 85
Hepatitis C, 80, 81, 85
Herpes, genital, **106**, **109**
Herpes simplex, 74, 76, 77, 81, 82, 85
Heterophyes heterophyes, 126
Histoplasmosis, 112
HIV, drugs for, **88**
chancroid, 108
crytosporidiosis, 123
cyclospora, 123
cytomegalovirus, 84
herpes simplex, 86
PCP pneumonia, 138
syphilis, 107
toxoplasmosis, 139
tuberculosis, 68
microsporidiosis, 136
HIV regimens, **95**
Hookworm infection, 128
HSV, 74, 76, 77, 81, 82, 85, **109**
Human immunodeficiency virus
see HIV
Hydatid cyst, 139
in pregnancy, 186
Hymenolepis nana, 139

Imipenem-cilastatin, 8
adverse effects, 150
dosage, 170
in pregnancy, 183
Imiquimod, 106, 108
Indinavir, **93**
adverse effects, 150
dosage, 170
in pregnancy, 188
indications, 68
Influenza, 75, 81, 83, 87
Interactions, drug
with fluconazole, 116
with itraconazole, 116
with ketoconazole, 117
with protease inhibitors, 68
with rifamycins, 67, 68
with voriconazole, 118
Interferon alfa, **79**
adverse effects, 150
dosage, 84, 85, 172
in pregnancy, 188
Iodoquinol
adverse effects, 150
in pregnancy, 186
indications and dosage, 120, 123, 124
Isoniazid, 14, 19
adverse effects, 69, 151
dosage, 72, 172
in pregnancy, 187
indications, **66**
Isospora belli, 128
Isosporiasis, 128
Itraconazole, **116**
adverse effects, 151
dosage, 111, 112. 113, 170
in pregnancy, 185
indications, 121
Ivermectin
adverse effects, 151
in pregnancy, 186
indications, 108, 121, 122, 123, 128, 129, 138

Kala-azar, 128
Kanamycin, 5
adverse effects, 69, 151
dosage, 73, 172
in pregnancy, 183
indications, 67

Ketoconazole, **117**
adverse effects, 151
dosage, 113, 172
in pregnancy, 185
indications, 103, 121
Klebsiella pneumoniae, 45

Lamivudine, **80, 89**
adverse effects, 151
dosage, i84, 172
in pregnancy, 188
Lassa fever, 82
Legionella, 49
Leishmaniasis, 128
Leprosy, 50
Leptospira, 52
Leptotrichia buccalis, 49
Leucovorin, 138, 140
Levamisole, 123
Levofloxacin, 13
adverse effects, 149
dosage, 73, 103, 104, 172
in pregnancy, 183
indications, 67, 99, 101
Lice, 129
Lincomycin, 14
adverse effects, 151
Lindane, in pregnancy, 186
Linezolid, 14
dosage, 172
in pregnancy, 184
Liposomal amphotericin B
adverse effects, 114
dosage, 162
Listeria monocytogenes, 44
Loa loa, 125
Lomefloxacin, 13
adverse effects, 149
dosage, 172
in pregnancy, 183
Lopinavir/ritonavir, **94**
adverse effects, 151
dosage, 172
in pregnancy, 188
Loracarbef, 10
adverse effects, 146
dosage, 172
in pregnancy, 182
Lung Fluke, 126
Lyme disease, 52
Lymphogranuloma venerum, 51, 103

Macrolides, 14
Malaria, 130
Malathion, 128
adverse effects, 151
in pregnancy, 186
Mansonella ozzardi, 125
Mansonella perstans, 125
Mansonella streptocerca, 126
MDRTB, **67**
Mebendazole
adverse effects, 151
in pregnancy, 186
indications, 121, 122, 123, 124, 125, 128, 139, 140, 141, 142
Mefloquine
adverse effects, 152
in pregnancy, 131, 145, 186
indications and dosage, 131, 134
Meglumine antimoniate
adverse effects, 152
indications and dosage, 128
Melarsoprol
adverse effects, 152
indications and dosage, 142
Melioidosis, 48
Meningitis, choice of antibacterials, **35**
Meningococcus, 43
Meropenem, 8
adverse effects, 152
dosage, 172
in pregnancy, 184
Metagonimus yokogawai, 126
Methenamines, 16
adverse effects, 152
dosage, 174
in pregnancy, 184
Methicillin, 17
adverse effects, 154

Methicillin-resistant staphylococci, 40
Methylbenzethonium, 129
Metorchis conjunctus, 126
Metronidazole, 16
  adverse effects 152
  dosage, 61, 104, 105, 174
  in pregnancy, 184, 186
  indications, 101, 102, 120, 123, 124, 127, 141
Miconazole
  adverse effects, 152
  dosage, 174
  in pregnancy, 185
  indications, 102, 121
Microsporidiosis, 136
Miltefosine
  indications and dosage, 128
Minocycline, 20
  adverse effects, 157
  dosage, 178
  in pregnancy, 184
Mobiluncus, 102
Moniliformis moniliformis, 136
Moraxella catarrhalis, 43
Morganella morganii, 46
Moxifloxacin, 13
  adverse effects, 149
  dosage, 73, 174
  in pregnancy, 183
MPC, 99
Mucopurulent cervicitis, **99**
Mucormycosis, 113
Mycobacterium avium complex, 50
Mycobacterium fortuitum
Mycobacterium kansasii, 50
Mycobacterium leprae, 50
Mycobacterium marinum, 50
Mycobacterium tuberculosis, 50, **66**
Mycoplasma genitalium, 99
Mycoplasma hominis, 101
Mycoplasma pneumoniae, 51

***N**aegleria species*, 121
Nafcillin, 17
  adverse effects, 154
  dosage, 174
  in pregnancy, 184
Nalidixic acid, 18
  adverse effects, 152
  dosage, 174
  in pregnancy, 184
Nanophyetus salmincola, 126
Necator americanus, 128
Neisseria gonorrhoeae, 43, **100**, **103**
Neisseria meningitidis, 43
Nelfinavir, **93**
  adverse effects, 152
  dosage, 174
  in pregnancy, 188
  indications, 68
Neomycin, 6, 120
  adverse effects, 153
  dosage, 61
Neomycin-gramicidin-polymyxin B
  dosage, 62
Neurosyphilis, 105
Nevirapine, **91**
  adverse effects, 153
  dosage, 174
  in pregnancy, 188
  indications, 68
NGU, 99
Niclosamide
  adverse effects, 153
  in pregnancy, 186
  indications and dosage, 139
Nifurtimox
  adverse effects, 153
  indications and dosage, 141
Nitazoxanide, 120, 123, 127
Nitrofurantoin, 16
  adverse effects, 153
  dosage, 174
  in pregnancy, 184
NNRTIs, 91
Nocardia, 50
Non-nucleoside reverse transcriptase inhibitors, **91**
Norfloxacin, 13
  adverse effects, 149
  dosage, 174
  in pregnancy, 183

NRTIs, 88
Nucleoside reverse transcriptase
  inhibitors, 88, **90**
Nystatin
  adverse effects, 153
  in pregnancy, 185

Octreotide, 136
Oesophagostomum bifurcum, 136
Ofloxacin, 13
  adverse effects, 149
  dosage, 62, 73, 103, 104, 174
  in pregnancy, 183
  indications, 99, 100, 101
Onchocerca volvulus, 126
Opisthorchis viverrini, 126
Orientia tsutsugamushi, 52
Ornidazole, 121
  adverse effects, 153
Ornithosis, 51
Oseltamivir, **81**
  adverse effects, 153
  dosage, 86, 174
  in pregnancy, 188
Oxacillin, 17
  adverse effects, 154
  dosage, 176
  in pregnancy, 184
Oxamniquine
  adverse effects, 153
  in pregnancy, 186
  indications and dosage, 138
Oxytetracycline, 20
  adverse effects, 157
  dosage, 178
  in pregnancy, 184

Papillomavirus, 108
Paracoccidioidomycosis, 113
Paragonimus westermani, 127
Parasitic infections, drugs for, **120**
Paromomycin
  adverse effects, 154
  in pregnancy, 186
  indications and dosage, 120, 123, 124, 127, 128
PAS, see Aminosalicylic acid
Pasteurella multocida, 49
Pathogens in specific organs, **22**
Pediculosis, **108**
Pediculus humanus, capitis, 129
Pegylated interferon alfa, 80
  adverse effects, 150
  dosage, 172
  in pregnancy, 188
Pelvic inflammatory disease, **101**, **104**
Penciclovir, **81**
  dosage, 85
Penicillin allergy, 36, 60
Penicillinase-resistant penicillins, 17
Penicillins, 17
  adverse effects, 154
  dosage, 62, 105, 176
  in pregnancy, 184
  indications, 107
Pentamidine
  adverse effects, 154
  in pregnancy, 186
  indications and dosage, 121, 122, 128, 137, 138, 141
Peptic ulcers, 45
Pepto-streptococcus, 42
Permethrin
  adverse effects, 155
  in pregnancy, 186
  indications, 108, 129, 138
PHMB, 120
Phthirus pubis, 108, 129
PID, 101, 104
Pinworm, 124
Piperacillin, 17
  adverse effects, 154
  dosage, 176
  in pregnancy, 184
Piperacillin-tazobactam, 17
  dosage, 176
  in pregnancy, 184
Piperazine, in pregnancy, 186
Plague, 50
Plasmodium falciparum, 130

Pleistophora sp., 136
Pneumococcus, 43
Pneumonia
  choice of antibacterials, **34**
Pneumocystis carinii, 137
Podofilox, 106
Podophyllin, 106
Polyhexamethylene biguanide, 120
Polymyxins, 18
  adverse effects, 155
Potassium iodide, 113
Praziquantel
  adverse effects, 155
  in pregnancy, 186
  indications and dosage, 126, 138, 139
Pregnancy
  antimicrobial safety, **182**
  antifungal use, **118**
  antiretrovirals, **94**
Primaquine
  adverse effects, 155
  in pregnancy, 186
  indications and dosage, 132, 133, 134, 138
Proguanil
  adverse effects, 155
  in pregnancy, 135
  indications and dosage, 130, 131, 134, 135
Propamidine isethionate, 120
Prophylaxis
  endocarditis, **64**
  fungal infections, 118
  patients with prosthetic joints, 60
  sexual assault, 109
  surgical site infection, **55**
Protease inhibitors, **92**
  and TB, 68
Proteus indole-positive, 46
Proteus mirabilis, 46
Proteus vulgaris, 46
Providencia rettgeri, 46
Providencia stuartii, 46
Pseudallescheriasis, 113
Pseudomonas, 100
Pseudomonas aeruginosa, 49
Pseudomonas mallei, 48
Pseudomonas pseudomallei, 49
Psittacosis, 51
Pyrantel pamoate
  adverse effects, 155
  in pregnancy, 186
  indications and dosage, 121, 122, 124, 128, 136, 141
Pyrazinamide, 18, 19
  adverse effects, 70, 155
  dosage, 72, 176
  in pregnancy, 187
  indications, **66**
Pyrethrins with piperonyl butoxide
  adverse effects, 155
  in pregnancy, 186
  indications, 129
Pyrimethamine
  adverse effects, 155
  in pregnancy, 186
  indications and dosage, 127, 139, 140
Pyrimethamine-sulfadoxine
  in pregnancy, 187
  indications and dosage, 130, 135

Q fever, 52
Quinacrine
  adverse effects, 155
  in pregnancy, 187
  indications and dosage, 127
Quinidine gluconate
  indictions and dosage, 133
Quinine
  adverse effects, 156
  in pregnancy, 187
  indications, 122, 130, 133
Quinolones, 18
Quinupristin/Dalfopristin, 18
  adverse effects, 156
  dosage 176
  in pregnancy, 184

Rat bite fever, 49
Relapsing fever, 52
Respiratory syncytial virus, 87
Rhodococcus equi, 51
Ribavirin, 79, **82**
  adverse effects, 156
  dosage, 85, 87, 176
  in pregnancy, 188
Rickettsia, 52
Rifabutin, 19
  adverse effects, 69, 156
  dosage, 72, 176
  in pregnancy, 187
  indications, 68
Rifamate, 68, 73
Rifampin, 14, 19
  adverse effects, 69, 156
  dosage, 72, 176
  in pregnancy, 187
  indications, **66**, 121
Rifapentine, 19
  adverse effects, 69, 156
  dosage, 72, 176
  in pregnancy, 187
Rifater, 67, 73
Rimantadine, **75**
  adverse effects, 156
  dosage, 86, 176
  in pregnancy, 188
Ritonavir, **93**
  adverse effects, 156
  dosage, 178
  in pregnancy, 188
  indications, 68
River Blindness, 125
Rocky Mountain spotted fever, 52
Roundworm, 122
RSV, 82, 87

Salmonella, 46
Salmonella typhi, 46
Sappinia diploidae, 121
Saquinavir, **93**
  adverse effects, 156
  dosage, 178
  in pregnancy, 188
  indication, 68
Sarcoptes scabiei, 108, 138
Scabies, **108**, 138
Schistosomiasis, 138
Sepsis, choice of antibacterials, **37**
Septata intestinalis, 136
Serratia, 47
Sexually transmitted diseases
  drugs for, **99**, **103**
Sheep liver fluke, 126
Shigella, 47
Sleeping sickness, 141
Sodium stibogluconate
  see Stibogluconate sodium
Southeastern Asian Liver Fluke, 126
Spectinomycin, 19
  adverse effects, 156
  dosage, 104, 178
  in pregnancy, 184
  indications, 101
Spiramycin
  adverse effects, 157
  indications and dosage, 140
Spirillum minus, 49
Spirochetes, 52
Sporotrichosis, 113
Staphylococcus aureus, 40
Staphylococcus epidermidis, 40
Stavudine, **88**
  adverse effects, 157
  dosage, 178
  in pregnancy, 188
Stenotrophomonas maltophilia, 49
Stibogluconate sodium
  adverse effects, 156
  indications and dosage, 128
Streptobacillus moniliformis, 49
Streptococcus bovis, 42
Streptococcus Group B, 42
Streptococcus pneumoniae, 42
Streptococcus pyogenes, 41
Streptococcus viridans, 42
Streptomycin, 6
  adverse effects, 70, 157
  dosage, 72, 178

in pregnancy, 184, 187
indications, 66
Strongyloides stercoralis, 138
Strongyloidiasis, 138
Sulbactam, 7
Sulfadiazine
indications and dosage, 121, 140
Sulfamethoxazole, 21
Sulfisoxazole, 15, 19
dosage, 178
Sulfonamides, 19
adverse effects, 157
in pregnancy, 184
Suramin
adverse effects, 157
in pregnancy, 187
indications and dosage, 141, 142
Surgery, antimicrobial prophylaxis, **55**
choice of drugs, **61**
Susceptibility tests, **27**
Syphilis, 52, **105**, **107**

Taenia saginata, 139
Taenia solium, 139
Tapeworm infection, 139
Tenofovir, **90**
adverse effects, 157
dosage, 178
in pregnancy, 188
Terbinafine, adverse effects, 157
Terconazole, indications, 102
Tetracyclines, 20
adverse effects, 157
dosage, 178
in pregnancy, 184
indictions, 123, 124, 130, 131
Thiabendazole
adverse effects, 158
in pregnancy, 187
indications and dosage, 122, 123, 138
Ticarcillin, 20
adverse effects, 154
dosage, 178
in pregnancy, 184
Ticarcillin-clavulanic acid, 20
adverse effects, 154
dosage, 178
in pregnancy, 184
Tinadazole
adverse effects, 158
indications and dosage, 102, 120, 121, 127, 140
Tioconazole, indications, 102
Tobramycin, 6
adverse effects, 158
dosage, 62, 178
in pregnancy, 185
Toxocariasis, 142
Toxoplasma gondii, 140
Toxoplasmosis, 140
TPE, 126
Trachipleistophora, 136
Trachoma, 51
Trench fever, 52
Treponema pallidum, 52, 105, **107**
Treponema pertenue, 52
Trichinella spiralis, 140
Trichinosis, 140
Trichloroacetic acid, 106
Trichomonas vaginalis, 141
Trichomoniasis, **102**, 105, 141
Trichostrongylus infection, 141
Trichuriasis, 141
Trichuris trichiura, 141
Triclabendazole
indications and dosage, 126
Trifluridine, 82
adverse effects, 158
dosage, 86
Trimethoprim, 20
adverse effects, 158
dosage, 178
in pregnancy, 185
indications, 137
Trimethoprim-sulfamethoxazole, 21
adverse effects, 158
dosage, 178
in pregnancy, 185
indications, 121, 122, 123, 124, 128, 137, 140

Trimetrexate
adverse effects, 158
indications and dosage, 137
Troleandomycin, 15
adverse effects, 158
Tropheryma whippelii, 51
Tropical Pulmonary Eosinophilia, 126
Trovafloxacin, 13
Trypanosomiasis, 141
Tuberculosis, drugs for, **66**
Tularemia, 48
TWAR, 51
Typhoid fever, 46
Typhus, 52
Ureaplasma urealyticum, 51, 99

Urethritis, nongonococcal, 99
Urinary tract infection,
choice of antibacterials, **39**

Vaginosis, **102**, 105
Valacyclovir, **82**
adverse effects, 159
dosage, 106, 178
dosage, 85, 86, 87
in pregnancy, 188
indications, 109
Valganciclovir, **83**
adverse effects, 159
dosage, 84, 180
in pregnancy, 188
Vancomycin, 21
adverse effects, 158
dosage, 61, 62, 63, 65, 180
in pregnancy, 185
indications, 55
Varicella, 74, 87
Vibrio cholerae, 50
Vibrio vulnificus, 50
Vidarabine, in pregnancy, 188
Viral infections, drugs for, **84**
Visceral larva migrans, 142
Vittaforma corneae, 136
VZV, 74, 87

Warts, genital, 106, **107**
West Nile virus, 82
Whipple's disease, 51
Whipworm, 141
Whooping cough, 47
Wolbachia, 125
Wuchereria bancrofti, 125

Yaws, 52
Yersinia enterocolitica, 47
Yersinia pestis, 50

Zalcitabine, **90**
adverse effects, 159
dosage, 180
in pregnancy, 188
Zanamivir, **83**
adverse effects, 159
dosage, 86, 180
in pregnancy, 188
Zidovudine, **88**
adverse effects, 159
dosage, 180
in pregnancy, 188
Zoster, 74, 87

NOTES

NOTES